ANXIOUS MAN

For Cali

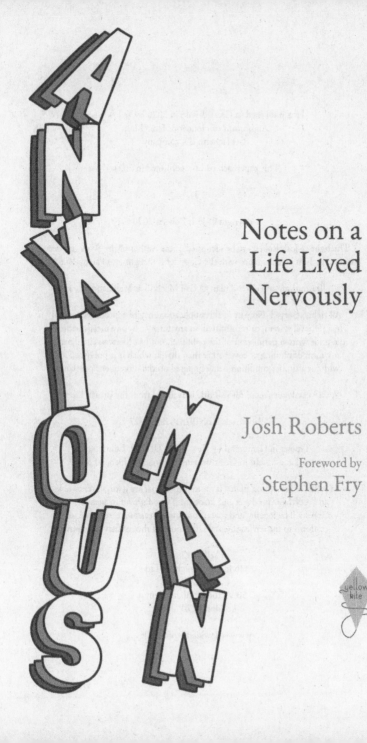

ANXIOUS MAN

Notes on a Life Lived Nervously

Josh Roberts

Foreword by
Stephen Fry

yellow
kite

First published in Great Britain in 2020 by Yellow Kite
An imprint of Hodder & Stoughton
An Hachette UK company

This paperback edition published in 2021

1

A CIP catalogue record for this title is available from the British Library

Paperback ISBN 9781529364927

Typeset in Garamond by Hewer Text UK Ltd, Edinburgh
Printed and bound in Great Britain by Clays Ltd, Elcograf S.p.A.

Hodder & Stoughton policy is to use papers that are natural, renewable
and recyclable products and made from wood grown in sustainable
forests. The logging and manufacturing processes are expected to
conform to the environmental regulations of the country of origin.

Yellow Kite
Hodder & Stoughton Ltd
Carmelite House
50 Victoria Embankment
London EC4Y 0DZ

www.yellowkitebooks.co.uk

CONTENTS

FOREWORD

THE WORLD IS getting used to the idea that all forms of
mental unease, distress, ill health and unhappiness are worth
talking about. That seems an absurd thing to have to write,
but we are an absurd species of course. Our contradictions
and confusions take so much getting used to that it is easier
to leave them to musicians, artists and neuroscientists to
illuminate or worry over while we compliment ourselves on
'getting on with living in the real world' – perhaps the great-
est delusion of them all. We know, for example, that income,
status, privilege and possessions do not sum to the condition
called Happiness, but we are bewildered and confounded
when we are inwardly miserable yet outwardly prospering.
We know that to be in a rut is undesirable, yet we are terrified of going 'off the rails'. But what are rails but inverted
ruts? We are mad in our refusal to understand that as a
species we are mad.

Of course, the horizontal sweep of such high words and
grand realisations does nothing to address the vertical

moments of misery and unhappiness that afflict so many of us without apparent reason. We have, at least, now reached a point where we are more comfortable in addressing the reality of mental health. We know, or should know, about various clinical conditions: mood disorders and personality disorders, for example. Thanks to all kinds of initiatives, thanks to individuals from princes to sporting heroes, we are aware of the scale and depth of the mental health crisis that has lain below the surface of society hidden and ashamed for so long. We have begun to talk about it, which is the first step. That step is always too small and always too slow, but nonetheless without it we cannot progress at all.

It is the daily experience of those out of the public eye whose stories most resonate, however. The experiences of people like . . . well, people like me in my flakey world of showbusiness and media attention, cocooned in celebrity and given permission to be eccentric, endearingly open and bravely unashamed – it is relatively easy for us to open up and while I am not going to writhe in apology or overdone modesty about the effect that this may have, I must be clear that it is without doubt easier for us. I suppose those in the public eye will always break cover first when coming out in matters like sexuality and health status, but it is the second wave of activists that matters. The second wave is made up of those whose experiences are not news or fodder for chat shows but which reflect much more accurately the life stories of the majority, out of the spotlight. The second wave includes those like Josh Roberts. *Anxious Man*, his magnificent account of a dizzying and dangerous descent into a turbulent and terrifying maelstrom of anxiety, is so truthful, bold, clear, candid and convincing that I read it in one breathless sitting. It connected with me, not because I – thanks heavens – suffer from exactly those kinds of destabilising terrors myself, but because I know so many people who do and who have not found a representative or a champion who can voice their condition. The bravura energy of his writing and the clarity, pain and wit with which his story is revealed are the guarantee of its authenticity and truth. This book, I am convinced, should be required reading for anyone who knows someone who might be going through the same overwhelming experience or might be going through it themselves.

And of course, if you do feel that you too are being taken over by such feelings then go and see a doctor as soon as you can and don't be put off until you are sure that he or she has taken you seriously.

Stephen Fry – Actor, Writer, Presenter

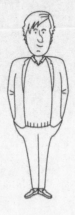

INTRODUCTION

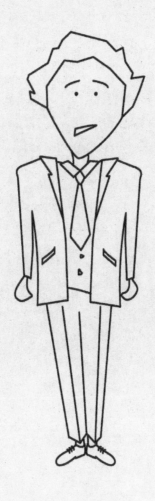

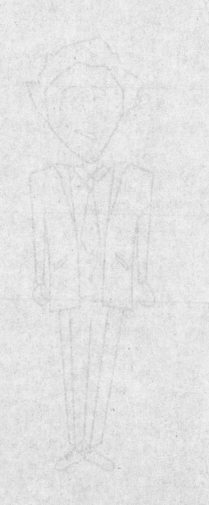

INTRODUCTION

FOUR YEARS AGO my mind collapsed.

It was all terribly sudden. One day I was a cheery, chirpy twenty-something, the next I was a hot mess of panic and tears. Eventually I was diagnosed with generalised anxiety disorder (GAD).

Since then I've been trying to get better, and learning to live my nervous life. Which is what this book is all about.

I'm going to tell you what it felt like to wake up one morning and realise that my mind was in free fall. I'm going to tell you why I think it happened to me. And, most importantly, I'm going to tell you what I've done to get better.

I'm afraid there will be moments of desperation and exhaustion. Those moments in the past few years when I've been in so deep, and the tide has been so strong, that it felt easier to just swim down.

But I can also promise moments of clarity. Those days when my mind has returned to its previous state. When my thoughts are clear. When my smile is broad. When I'm happy, and peaceful, and loving, and being loved.

More than anything, there will be the relief at realising, as I am starting to realise, that all this isn't forever. That clouds lift, days break. That, over time, the periods of mental convulsion become shorter and the distances between them grow larger.

But before we begin, some caveats:

1. Every person and every brain and every mental health problem is different

My experience is personal to me, and will likely differ from yours or that of your girlfriend/boyfriend/friend/sister/brother/father/pet hamster. And that's fine.

Through many hours of chit-chat with therapists, I've come to understand that simple, sweeping categorisations for mental health problems are counterproductive. They're clunky and blunt.

In reality, mental health is much more like one of those lunches you have on a hot holiday, a 'picky picky' as my mother would say. On my plate there are some nice big slices of anxiety, a few leaves of depression (for crunch) and a good hunk of obsessive compulsive disorder (OCD) to mop it all up with.

The meze selection of others might look different to mine, but I'd be surprised if we didn't have some picky bits in common. I'd be even more surprised if what has helped me doesn't help others. At the very least, I hope it will make folks realise that they're not alone.

2. I am a middle-class, heterosexual, white man

And I'm privileged in a million other ways beyond that – I've got supportive and generous parents, and kind and funny friends. I got a fancy education, and I've had well-paying jobs. I don't apologise for any of this, but I am aware of it; I know how lucky I have been.

It's important that you know that I know this. Because later on you might find yourself thinking, 'Just pull yourself together you silly posho' and, while I completely understand that, it's important to know that mental ill health can affect everyone. It doesn't discriminate. It doesn't care where you live or what your dad does for a living. It's an everyman kinda thing, like spaghetti Bolognese or IKEA.

3. I am unfixable

Over the past couple of years I have spoken to tons of friends, friends of friends and colleagues. Their problems and the questions they ask have varied greatly. But common to them all is this notion of being 'fixed'.

'How long does it last?' they might ask. Or, 'You're fixed now, right?'

No, I'm not.

Definitely, I'm a lot, lot better than I was three years ago. But I still have good days and horrible weeks. I still worry and panic. I still have moments when I hate myself. I still wish this hadn't happened to me. I'm still a bit broken.

I'd hate for you to think that mental health problems have beginnings, middles and ends. They don't. They're untidy, jumbled and chaotic. Today I'm good. Tomorrow I could be awful. What's important is that, while at the start I was completely helpless in the face of the bad days, now I have a plan.

Oh, and one more thing. Obviously, I'm not a scientist or mathematician, so if you're expecting lots of pie charts, or those ones with boxes and whiskers, then I'm afraid you're going to be disappointed. There will be a few little visual explainers, but nothing too complicated.

If all that sounds good, then I suggest we get cracking.

ANATOMY OF A BREAKDOWN

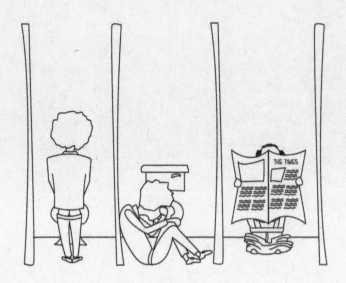

ANATOMY OF A BREAKDOWN

IT'S A FUNNY business, crying in the loos at work.

The usual form when crying is to let your body do whatever it wants. You allow yourself to contort and push and twist. You force the emotion out. You squeeze and squirm and shudder.

But you can't do any of that in the loos at work. You must stay completely frozen and silent, so as to avoid giving the game away. You must keep your legs still and snuffle your sniffles with a fist full of loo roll. You must remember to do a 'phantom flush' lest Gary from Accounts in the adjacent cubicle smells a rat. After all, as every ex-public school boy knows, the only thing worse than crying in the bogs is someone else knowing that you're crying in the bogs.

So there I'd sit on the cold marble floor, head in one hand, phone blinking with fresh emails in the other, hoping that at some point the torment in my head would pass.

For nearly two years this sorry sight was part of my daily routine. Some days I could manage a few hours at my desk before my first trip to toilet cubicle two. Other days it was more urgent. Often it was the first thing I did on reaching the office. I couldn't stop it, I couldn't control it and I couldn't bear it. I just had to cry.

It all started after I went to a party – *that fucking party* – a farewell bash for some friends who were moving to South Africa. Not a particularly big party, mind you. Nor, as it happened, a very good one. And I'd actually been quite well behaved. Drunk enough to dance, sure, but not much more.

So, as I lay atop the bed covers fully clothed the next morning, light searing in through my lazily uncurtained windows, I felt a deep sense of injustice. I hadn't expected any hangover at all, let alone one of this intensity. And it *was* intense. Assessing the damage, I ran through my usual Sunday morning checklist:

- Half drunk bottle of Peroni on the bedside table? Check.
- Headache? Check.
- Nausea? Check.
- Dry, itchy eyes? Check.

All standard stuff, except it wasn't. Something was amiss. Something about this particular hangover wasn't right.

Why is my chest tight? Why am I beginning to sweat? Why is my vision blurred? Why can't I breathe? Why is my heart pounding? Why won't it stop? What is happening? Why is my heart thumping like this? Fuck I'm dying. Fuck I'm going to have a heart attack. FUCK. FUCK.

I'M FUCKING DYING. I'M ABOUT TO FUCKING DIE!

It came in waves. Inexorable waves of panic, which would surge up from just underneath my solar plexus and ripple out across my body. I didn't, or maybe couldn't, move. I just lay there, frozen in fear, mouth open, eyes fixed on the ceiling, waiting for the next convulsion, assuming that at some point it would be curtains for me.

I stayed like that for 10 minutes before, finally, the waves began to subside. Although they never fully subsided. For the rest of the day, every 30 minutes or so, there'd be another judder, another crack of panic. My chest would tighten, my heart would thump and the singular mental terror of imminent death would return. It didn't follow any schedule or rhythm. The claxon of consternation would sound without any warning. I remember trying to make lunch when – WHACK – a new hurricane of panic arrived. I dropped the plate, crumpled to the floor, closed my eyes and screamed.

I tried everything to make the feelings of nervousness go away – showering, eating, exercising – but to no avail. When evening arrived, I even tried drinking a beer. Actually, I tried drinking a few. But that didn't work either. If anything, my mind whirred even faster than before. I could feel my chest constricting with every cold, fizzy gulp.

I didn't sleep a wink that night. I tried to, of course. But sleep is like getting an erection – the more you think about it, the less likely it becomes. 'If only I could sleep,' I said to myself. 'I need to sleep.'

It took forever for Monday morning to arrive. I tossed, I turned, I stared demonically at the alarm clock. During one surge of anxiety I very nearly called an ambulance, but managed to talk myself out of it. My situation was already pretty embarrassing, and having other people know about it would only make it worse.

I can't tell you how I got to work that morning, but somehow I did.

'Good weekend?' asked my smiley colleague, Lily, as I approached my desk.

'Not really, Lil',' I said staring emptily ahead.

'Are you all right?' she asked. 'You look like shit.'

Or at least I think that's what she said. If I'm honest, she'd lost me at 'Good weekend?' I'd stopped listening, and started panicking.

Without saying another word, without even taking my coat off, I made for the toilets, crashed into a cubicle, slammed the door shut, fell to the floor and began crying. Not sobbing or weeping, but full-on, visceral, abdominal crying. That's how the crying started. That's how it all started. That's how I broke down.

Panic stations!

If you've never experienced a panic attack I suspect it all sounds a bit wishy-washy. Like the sort of thing that wouldn't have existed a hundred years ago. They'd have called it a 'funny turn' or a 'momentary hysteria'. Wet

---

flannels would have been sought, leeches would have been applied.

Unfortunately, panic attacks are real things. They're not dangerous, but they are real and they are terrifying.

For me the physical stuff comes first. My heart pumps harder than before, harder than I think it can. The muscles across my chest tighten, and tighten, and tighten, until my breath becomes short and shallow. Sweat melts out of every pore. I'm dizzy. My eyes can't focus.

Some people can stand up while they have a panic attack. I can't. I wither and collapse to the floor, or into a chair, or onto a bed. My body is just too focused on panicking to do anything else.

Accompanying the physical terror is the mental one. There's only one thought in my mind when I'm having a panic attack – 'I'm about to die!' screams the voice inside my head. Over, and over, and over again at voice-cracking, ear-splitting volume.

It's how I imagine a pilot feels in the moments before a plane crash. I'm about to die and there's nothing I can do to stop it. I have no way, no mechanism, of regaining control. It's over. It's about to happen. I'm going to expire. In a few moments I'll slam into the ground and everything will go black.

I can't be with other people when I'm having a panic attack. I don't want to be seen, and I don't want to see. I don't need support or reassurance. I need it to be over. I need it to pass. I need it to be 10 minutes into the future, right now.

I've known Guy for nearly 15 years. As well as being an incredible GP, he's also my friend's dad. And a cool dude – one of those parents who you actually look forward to seeing. Over the years he's patched up loads of my mates. Always in confidence, with a smile and with an answer. After two weeks of crying in the toilets at work, I booked an appointment, moped into his surgery and sat down silently.

'What seems to be the problem?' he said.

I told him everything. I told him about the party a fortnight ago. I told him about the Sunday morning panic attack, the crying in the loos, the fact that I couldn't stop worrying.

'What exactly are you worrying about?' he asked.

Everything. I was worrying about everything. It wasn't just a fear of immediate death any more. It had moved on. It had evolved from a series of finite panic attacks into a continuous, all-pervasive nervousness. A fear of fear. A worry about worry – an obsessive and involuntary one. As soon as my brain came up with something new to think – like what to wear to work or what to have for tea – the anxious thoughts would arrive.

'Never mind all that,' would come the interruption, 'you're about to have another panic attack and this time it'll be even worse than before.'

'Why has it taken you two weeks to see a doctor?' asked Guy.

It hadn't. In fact, Guy's was the sixth medical opinion I'd received. Although his was the only one that made sense. The others – the three different A&E doctors and two GPs – just thought I was being a bit silly. It was a hangover gone wrong, they said. I just needed to rest, to get some sleep, and everything would go back to normal.

'But I can't sleep,' I told them. 'I haven't slept for days.'

'Sorry,' they said, 'there's not much we can do.'

Guy did a few simple tests. Put your arm in this, look into that, breathe into this until you're puffed out. That sort of thing. Which, it turns out, is a standard quack tactic – run a few tests to make them think that you're investigating, then diagnose them with what you already knew it was.

'Have you ever heard of something like this before?' I said. 'I'm terrified.'

'Josh,' he said calmly and confidently, 'you have an anxiety disorder.'

It was the first time in my life that I'd been diagnosed with something. Unless you count conjunctivitis or a verruca (but I'm fairly sure you don't). Certainly I'd never had anything that came with a 'long-term management plan' or its own charity.

It was an odd feeling; a bizarre blend of relief that I wasn't the first to go through what I was experiencing, and alarm that I had got *something*. Something that could get better, stay the same or, God forbid, get worse. It was inside me, squatting in my brain. It could leave quickly and quietly after a few days, or it could be there forever. Maybe I'd be like this for the rest of my life. Maybe it would kill me.

I'm not being melodramatic, by the way – it could have killed me. Being a man under 50, I was already in the high-risk category for suicide. With this diagnosis that risk went up several notches.

Guy prescribed me with a Valium-type pill for use in emergencies and referred me to a CBT (cognitive behavioural therapy) therapist down the road.

'It'll get better,' he said. 'It'll take some work, but it will get better.'

I'd love to say that over the following few days I started the fightback, but that would be a lie. Instead I did what most people do when they're diagnosed with something: I talked about it incessantly, and googled the shit out of it.

The latter was a terrible idea (isn't it always?). I started out on the NHS website with its lovely, publicly funded, balanced and impartial advice. But that wasn't any good because it didn't tell me exactly what I wanted (i.e. that I would be completely fixed very quickly). So I cast the net a little wider, and very quickly found myself in the weird and woeful world of mental health forums. What fresh hell that was. Don't get me wrong – I love the Internet. If anything, I love it too much. It's just not very good at fixing mental health problems. Trawling the Internet to cure an anxiety disorder is like trying to extinguish a fire with petrol, or like trying to save a drowning person with a lead lifebelt, or whichever laboured metaphor you prefer. The point is, far from making me better, ingesting other people's misery made me much, much worse. It only gave me more things to worry about. Maybe, like @Meera_P4tel, I'd develop an eating disorder, too. Or I could become addicted to sleeping pills like @WilmaWondes. Or I could acquire a substance abuse problem like @MagicMark21.

Welcome to the Mental Health Muppets Forum!

The place where well-meaning pseudo-therapists and malevolent trolls come together to make your problem worse!

Please register to comment.

Thread: **Help! I think I have a problem.**

@Jimbob2340 Member: Posts: 1

hey guys. I'm a 24-year-old male. I had my first panic attack and I'm feeling really nervous the whole time about nothing in particular. Been like this for like a week. Will it get better?

@NiceKnowItAll Member: Posts: 42,567

sounds like you've got Generalised Anxiety Disorder. I've had it for 4 years. I'm much better now but it takes time to heal. Have you seen a doctor? Fingers are crossed for you.

@PessimistTroll Guest: Posts: 5

I agree with @NiceKnowItAll you've got GAD. You'll never get better. Mine is worse than ever. you will probs kill yourself.

@Jimbob2340 Member: Posts: 2

Thanks guys. I guess I'll see a doctor. Wish me luck!

@Trump4Pres_21 Member: Posts: 53

People like @Jimbob2340 make me sick. You are clearly very weak. You snowflakes need to man up!

The weeks that followed my diagnosis were exhausting. I ricocheted around, physically drained, but mentally wired. I had no plan at this stage beyond 'living'. I was at the mercy of the anxiety. It decided when I could sleep, what I could eat, how often I could see my friends. Sometimes it would allow me the odd smile or enjoyable trip to the cinema, but otherwise its leash was extremely tight. Just as I'd start to get excited about something, or even suggest that I was enjoying myself, the anxiety would call me to heel. 'There's no point in looking forward to the weekend,' it would say. 'You'll be nervous the whole time so there's no chance you'll enjoy it.' Sometimes I would challenge the thoughts, but often I just went with them. It was easier that way.

Outwardly I don't think much changed. I didn't lose any weight (sadly) or hair (thankfully), and I didn't call in sick to work. I must have been pretty weird at work though, dashing off to the loos, suddenly going silent in meetings, but never enough that my colleagues suspected something was up. I never cried openly or broke down in front of them, or anything juicy like that. In fact, thinking about it, I've only ever properly broken down in front of one person, my poor flatmate Adriana. It happened very early on when she came home from a work trip and found me hunched on the kitchen floor whispering 'I'm so fucked' over and over again. Not what she needed after a 10-hour flight back from India. She was lovely about it, of course.

It's difficult to say exactly how long this first 'phase' lasted. Six months, maybe. Six months – 180 days – of sheer, unchanging, obsessive, involuntary, intrusive worry. McDonald's used to advertise their 24-hour restaurants with the slogan 'If you're up, we're up', and it was like that with my anxiety. It was there *all the time*: from the moment my eyes opened, to the exact second I closed them.

'I won't be able to eat because I'll be nervous', 'My girl-friend will dump me because I'll always be nervous', 'I won't be able to sleep because I'll be nervous', 'I'm going to get fired because I'll be nervous' . . . Worry, worry, worry. It was relentless. It was exhausting. It was, speaking plainly, shite.

WORRYING ABOUT WORRYING

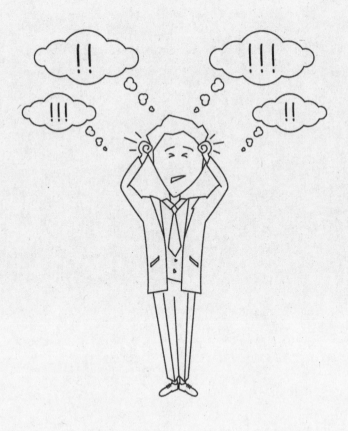

WORRYING ABOUT WORRYING

'SHOULD' IS A miserable word.

It's not a fun word or a word of pleasure. It's dull and dutiful. It's a word of obligation, burden and boredom. 'We *should* change our gas supplier', 'She *should* dump him', 'I *should* delete my Internet search history.'

More than that, though, 'should' is also a very dangerous word. In fact, for the depressed, anxious and obsessive, it's the most malevolent word in the English language.

I've suffered greatly at the hands of 'should'. It's the key ingredient for most of my anxious thoughts. Just as omelettes require eggs and bread requires flour, my anxiety depends on a healthy supply of 'shoulds': I *should* be happier, I *should* be enjoying myself, I *should* stop worrying, I *should* have slept better, I *should* be fulfilled at work, I *should* want sex the whole time . . . And so on.

'Should' creates expectation – expectation that I've got no hope of reaching – and that causes me to worry.

But it doesn't stop there. For 'normal' people it would. They'd be content with worrying about a missed expectation.

I'm not, my brain isn't. I go one step further. I begin to worry about that worry. 'I should have slept better' becomes 'I'm never going to enjoy life because I'll always be worrying about not sleeping.'

The transition from simple to compound worries is often extremely subtle, as well as being completely involuntary and, natch, totally obsessive. The thoughts just whirl and whirl around my head. The more I try to push them away, the faster and harder they return. Maybe I can sneak in the occasional mental ramble or the odd flight of cognitive fancy. But, if I do, it doesn't last long. Usually after a minute or so the school bell rings, the daydream evaporates and the inexorable focus on worrying, and worrying about worrying, returns.

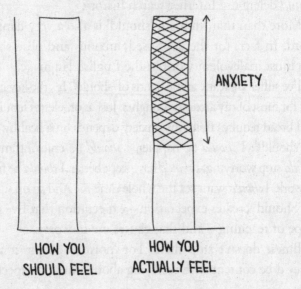

'SHOULD' WORRIES

ANXIETY

HOW YOU
SHOULD FEEL

HOW YOU
ACTUALLY FEEL

It's the same with the sensorimotor stuff.

For 26 years I had taken unconscious, sensorimotor exertions like breathing or blinking for granted. I could swallow like a champ, breathe like a boss. I had the best hypothalamus in the business.

After my breakdown – after *that fucking party* – that all changed. Suddenly I became hyper aware of the automatic functions of my brain. I was deeply alive to the depth of my breath, the pattern of my blinking, the mechanics of my swallowing. I developed an intense fear of getting something in my eye or stuck in my throat. I worried endlessly about forgetting to inhale or the idea of my heart stopping.

Of course, the awareness and worries themselves were tiring and debilitating. But, more than that, just as with 'shoulds', my mind went further and added a final, additional anxious flourish: 'You're never going to be happy because you'll always be worrying about breathing.'

Just writing these thoughts down now, I can see how obviously bizarre, so clearly silly, they are. But at the time I really bought into them. I believed them. I saw their logic. I found evidence to support them. They weren't invented anxious bullshit – they were *true*.

In contrast, I always suspected that my third group of anxious thoughts – the ego dystonic ones – *were* bullshit. Although that didn't stop me worrying about them too.

Ego dystonic thoughts are thoughts that we find distressing because they're inconsistent with the rest of our personalities. Loads of people get them. 'I could jump in front of that train' is a common one. As is 'I could open the plane door while we're flying' or 'I could drive the car onto the pavement.' Often they're sexual in nature: 'I could be gay' perhaps, or 'I could be attracted to my own child.'

Of course, deep down it's obvious that these thoughts are untrue, but often just having them is enough to send people into a spin. 'I've had a thought that I could be a sex pest, therefore I am one' is how the warped logic goes.

Interestingly, some experts I have spoken to have described a subtle, almost osmotic, relationship between common 'ego dystonic' thoughts and the news agenda of the day. Most recently, people have been presenting with worries about committing terrorist atrocities. They're not worrying because they are a terrorist; they're simply worrying because they had the thought. 'I could do something awful' is taken as evidence that they will.

My own ego dystonic thoughts are mostly about physical stuff. Not jumping in front of a train or out of planes, but things like 'I could stab myself with that knife' or 'I could break that glass and shove it in my eye.' From time to time I get social ones, too. I've sat through countless meetings thinking 'I could scream CUNT at the top of my voice.' And when I meet people's babies or children, my mind will imagine punching them in the face. It's the same when a cyclist cuts me up. On reflection, I'm not sure that has anything to do with my condition.

I've never followed through with any of these thoughts, of course. But that's not the point. The point is that ego dystonic intrusions represent a seed of worry that, in my anxious brain, quickly germinates and flourishes. 'I could swallow those nails' transmutes into 'I'm never going to enjoy life as I'll always be worrying about swallowing those nails.' It's frightening, annoying and exhausting.

There are subtle differences in the ways in which the three types of anxious thoughts – the 'shoulds', the sensorimotor and the ego dystonic – present themselves. 'Shoulds' usually require a run-up. It takes time for my mind to concoct a really potent, unachievable expectation. And even longer to begin worrying about it. 'I should be happier' wasn't dreamt up in a day, and neither was 'I'm never going to enjoy life because I'll constantly be worrying about not being happy.'

The sensorimotor and ego dystonic ones are much more immediate. They're the tiger sharks of the anxious mind – they're born fully formed, dangerous and ready to kill. I can be quite happily pottering about, reading a paper or writing another complaint email to the council ('Re: Noisy Neighbours') when – SLAM – I'm suddenly terrified: 'Fuck, I'm conscious of breathing' or 'I could smash that bottle into my face.'

Others have told me that their anxieties are triggered; that there are certain situations or events that set them off. Maybe someone says something or they see something on the telly that stimulates the intrusive thoughts. It doesn't work like that for me. For me it's totally random. As well as being completely involuntary.

I can't stop the execrable little buggers popping into my head. I can't stop them whirring around incessantly. And I certainly can't force them out. They're beyond my control, outside my purview. Which is an important point. It's what management consultants would call a 'key takeaway' or the 'take-home' or the 'take me out'. Here it is: *I can't stop myself from worrying, it just happens.*

I can no more stop the thoughts in my head than I can stop it snowing, or Tuesdays. I *can* influence how I react to the thoughts in my head (and we'll see how later), but I can't prevent them arriving. That's decided elsewhere, by something much more complex and clever than me. You could call it God, or you could call it random chance. Either way, I don't get to decide my thoughts.

The reason I stress this is because people who haven't had mental health problems often think that it's all voluntary. For them, being depressed or anxious or obsessive-compulsive is a choice. They reckon it's optional, elective. 'Cheer up' they say, or 'do try to stop worrying', or 'just snap out of it', as if I haven't tried that. As if they're expecting me to respond with 'Holy shit, Greg! What a brilliant idea! I'll just stop worrying, then I won't have this anxiety disorder!' Can you imagine using the same sentiments with physical health? It would be absurd. 'Do try not to have heart disease', or 'Still, plenty of reasons not to be asthmatic.' I can't opt out of anxiety any more than I can opt out of hay fever. Capeesh?

At the start, the anxious thoughts would occur constantly, but in isolation. I would spend a week agonising about a worry to do with breathing. Followed by a fortnight on a 'should'. And maybe a few days panicking about stabbing myself in the neck. After a few months that changed. Slowly my brain started to combine the different types of worry into new, stronger alloys. Thus a worry about eating glass became evidence that I would never sleep. Or not loving my girlfriend, Cali, enough meant that I would end up killing someone. And so on. The more complex and interdependent the worry, the more terrifying I found it. Piffling little grass snakes became a six-headed Hydra. The tangles of worry grew larger and tighter.

It was like that for the first year – constant, unstoppable worry, and worry about worry. Then two things happened. Firstly I started to get terribly, terribly down. And secondly I began to behave differently. The thoughts in my head made me do stuff and *not* do stuff. The obsessions in my mind compelled me to do certain things.

A MEZE OF MISERY

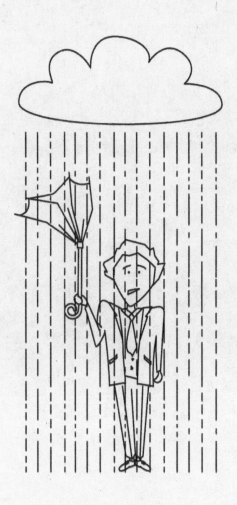

A MEZE OF MISERY

WITHOUT DOUBT, THE depression was the scariest.

The anxiety was frightening, maddening and exhausting. But the depression was worse. At least through the anxious episodes I wanted to get better. During the depressive ones I didn't. I couldn't. I couldn't force myself to exercise, or see friends, or breathe. I couldn't muster the energy to get better. And this, combined with the fact that I knew how depression ends, made it terrifying.

Depression and anxiety make odd, but extremely common bedfellows. Odd because, to me at least, they're polar opposites. Anxiety is a heightened, hot, intense state of being. It's frenzied and scatty. My mind fizzes and whirrs. It's a manic, nervous energy, but there is at least some energy. Depression is none of those things. It's the opposite. It's the absence of feeling. It's not sadness, it's nothingness. It's total apathy. It's cold and dank – a lead dressing gown, a damp, suffocating pillow over my face. The world is only grey and cold. Everything is shit.

I've had countless mini-episodes of depression and two big ones. The short ones last a day, the longer ones about two weeks. Regardless of the duration, though, the thoughts are always the same. Or rather the *thought* is always the same: 'Why am I so fucking useless?' As with the anxious thoughts, this depressive one comes involuntarily and obsessively. *Why am I so fucking useless?* Occasionally I'll introduce a snippet of evidence to prove that it's true. *I didn't sleep last night because I'm so fucking useless.* But mostly, I don't need to. *Why am I so fucking useless?* Mostly, it's just obvious. *Why am I so fucking useless?*

When I'm anxious I can do other things. I can function, and sometimes I can function pretty well. When I'm depressed I can't. Usually I just lie on the bed, stare at the ceiling and marinate in my own misery. In fact, just last month Cali found me sitting in the car, engine off, staring aimlessly ahead. I'd been in B&Q buying wall plugs (sexy, right?) when the depression hit. With no warning, this huge wall of apathy just slammed into me, right there in aisle four. Somehow, I made it through the checkout and managed to drive home.

'How long have you been here?' Cali asked me as I wound down the window.

'Oh, only a couple of minutes,' I lied. Judging by the clock in the car it had been at least an hour. And I'd left the fucking wall plugs in B&Q. *Why am I so fucking useless?*

The first big depressive episode was the closest I've ever come to killing myself. The second time I had some object-ivity – I'd lived through a bad patch and had some sense that it could get better. That wasn't the case with the first big low. I had no way of seeing beyond the despair. I'd just lie on the bed, or sit in a chair, and let the apathy and self-hatred wash over me. I thought about suicide quite a bit. On nights when I couldn't sleep, I'd imagine how I'd do it, and what it would feel like. I'd imagine my funeral, guessing at who would attend, and what they'd wear. I'd picture my father's quiet anguish, my mother's tears, my brothers, Cali crying as her friends Vicky and Laura consoled her. A common response when someone commits suicide is 'How selfish. Why didn't they think of their friends and family?' Let me assure you, when you're that down, when you're that close to death, your friends and family are *all you think about*. It's just that sometimes they're not enough. Sometimes people sink so low that not even their loved ones can save them.

That's how it was for my mate Max. Unlike me, he actually tried to go through with it. Not that I knew it at the time. Back then, I, like most of Max's mates, just thought he'd had a car crash. Now I know it was much more tragic than that. He was driving home from work at Christmas time and just decided, right there on the M1, that enough was enough. He's better now. Much better, thank God.

Initially, my weird behaviour was well-intentioned. It was born out of positivity, out of a willingness to get better. What happened was that about a month or so after the breakdown I had this marvellous idea to make two lists: one of things that made my anxiety better, and one of things that made it worse.

The idea being that if I could just eliminate the bad stuff, and do more of the good, then my anxiety would disappear. Sounds logical, right?

The lists were quite detailed. I'd start by jotting down my nervousness on a scale of 0 to 10 – with 0 being a Caribbean holiday and 10 being unbearable and unthinkable worry. Then I'd record the current circumstances (time of day, weather, work/home, etc.), and have a rummage through the previous 24 hours. Did I go to the gym yesterday? Did I drink caffeine in the afternoon? Did I eat dinner too late?

Having mapped my anxiety, the next step was to begin changing my behaviour. Whenever I thought I'd identified a bad thing, I did it less, and when I found a positive, I did it more. In fact, I did it obsessively.

Within weeks I'd developed a long and continually evolving list of rules within which I lived my life. I couldn't drink booze or coffee, for example. I couldn't eat chocolate or red meat. I couldn't see friends on Sundays, or see Cali on Tuesdays. I couldn't play five-a-side ever, or walk to work on Thursdays. I couldn't have meetings in the morning, and had to exercise in the evening (every day). I had to walk a minimum of 10,000 steps a day, and take vitamin supplements, and do my breathing exercises. By the end, the list of rules and regulations was so long that it was pretty much all I had. The vast majority of my day would be spent simply servicing the compulsions. There wasn't much room for anything else in my life.

15 rules for an anxiety-free life*

- Never drink alcohol.
- Never drink caffeine.
- Never eat chocolate.
- Never eat red meat.
- Never see friends on Sundays.
- Never spend any time alone.
- Never read, watch or listen to anything related to anxiety.
- Never have meetings in the morning.
- Never go to bed before 10pm.
- Exercise every day.
- Drink five litres of water per day.
- Walk a minimum of 10,000 steps per day.
- Take vitamin supplements.
- Always sleep with a fan.
- Never admit to feeling anxious.

The great irony was that I'd started doing all this stuff to make the anxiety go away, but, in reality, it only made the quagmire deeper. It became yet another thing to worry about. 'I haven't done my 10,000 steps today so I'll be worried for the rest of my life.'

The big one was spending time alone. The lists were clear on that – whenever I spent time on my own it got worse. So

* Note: all of these are bullshit.

the obvious answer, the natural compulsion, was to avoid solitude. So I did.

I started timing my morning routine to coincide perfectly with my flatmate's, to ensure that I didn't commute alone. I'd wait to hear her door crack open and then leg it into the corridor.

'Are you leaving soonish?' I'd ask with faux nonchalance. 'I could walk with you to the station.'

'Isn't that the wrong direction for you?' she would respond.

'Oh, it's not too bad. I rather like the walk.'

Evenings were fastidiously planned to make sure that I wouldn't be alone. I booked dinners, took up cycling and even started tutoring GCSE Maths to underprivileged children (I know, I do too much). Often I'd double-book myself as insurance against being cancelled on. It meant that I quite often had to let friends down, but that was a price worth paying to prevent me being on my tod.

Monday evenings were a problem. No one wants to do anything on a Monday. They're all too busy 'having a chilled one mate . . . big weekend'. Humph. At one stage the Monday evening dilemma got so bad that I even signed up for a Spanish class at the local community centre. It was unbearable and I didn't last long. Or, rather, *no duré mucho*.

There were moments when my obsessions and their accompanying compulsions got pretty bad. Particularly in the area of sleep. I used to do all sorts in pursuit of 40 winks. I tried not going to bed until 2am. I tried not going to bed after 9pm. I tried taking supplements. I tried reading (but nothing too exciting). I tried herbal teas, drinking water, not drinking water. I tried lying on the floor. I tried going to the loo after turning out the lights. I tried not turning out the lights. I tried podcasts. I bought a bedroom fan. And on, and on, and on.

By the end there must have been 20 things I *had* to do before shutting my eyes. It was torture. And not just for me – poor Cali also suffered. In the four years that we've been together we've only ever argued about two things: my bizarre sleeping rituals and whether you put the milk in first.

'You don't understand,' I'd say, 'I have to do this stuff if I'm going to sleep.'

'What about me?' she'd respond (entirely fairly). 'It's impossible to relax with you rushing around the room switching on fans and flushing the loo.'

Throughout all my 'troubles' I've always tried to be forgiving of people saying the wrong things. We live in easily offended times, and I'm loath to join the ranks of the perpetually wronged. So I try not to cringe when I overhear 'I'm so *depressed* now that *Game of Thrones* has finished.' And I try not to bristle when someone says 'Bottomless brunches give me serious *anxiety*.'

But I'm afraid I crack with the obsessive-compulsive ones. I can't help it; I'm compelled to intervene (pun intended). No sooner has someone launched into their 'I'm a bit OCD' routine than I find myself lecturing them on how serious and enfeebling a condition OCD can be.

It wasn't for me, though. For me it was only ever a support act – a really fucking annoying one – for my anxiety and depression. But I've met people whose lives have been utterly devastated by obsessions and compulsions. I know a girl who didn't leave the house for two years, such was the intensity of her contamination fears. I know a man who had to quit his job because he was so scared of harming his colleagues. I know another man who had to cut himself to sleep. Awful, I know. And worth bearing in mind the next time Carol from HR starts yammering on about her sock drawer, or how she has to check the front door.

It was rare that I experienced anxiety, depression and OCD on their own. Usually they were interwoven and interdependent. I think of it in terms of Destiny's Child (stay with me). Definitely anxiety was the lead singer, the Beyoncé, of the band. But, she wouldn't be anything without the support of Kelly (depression) and Michelle (OCD). From time to time Beyoncé would step back and allow one of the others to take the lead. But everyone knew that she was still in charge. She was the one driving the concert; she was the most powerful vocalist.

Doubtless for others it's different. I'm sure some folks just get the OCD, or only have the depression. Either way, as my granny would say, 'Everyone has their cross to bear.' Or, rather, everyone has their meze to munch.

I CAN'T GET NO SLEEP

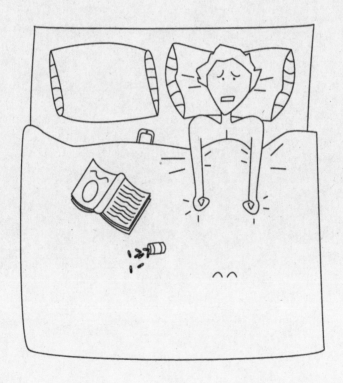

I CAN'T GET NO SLEEP

IN MY EXPERIENCE there are two types of sleepless nights.

The first are what I call the 'non-starters'. These are the evenings where I know from the outset that sleep won't be visiting me. I'll still go through the rigmarole of getting ready for bed (showering, brushing teeth, etc.); I just know that it's futile. Sometimes I don't even bother turning out the light. And if I do, it's usually only for a while. For 20 minutes or so I'll try desperately to think of things to fill my mind. I'll think about the day just gone, or run through my plans for the next one. But at some point the words 'I'm never going to sleep tonight' will pop into my head and, from that moment, the battle is lost. A small wave of anxiety will pass through my body, my breathing will shorten, my eyes will open. The sheets, once cool and crisp, are, in a moment, hot and clammy. Sometimes I toss and turn, sometimes I get up. Usually, I just turn the lights back on and lie there in silent frustration wishing for morning.

'Sleepless' isn't perhaps the right word for the second kind of insomniac night because there are snatched moments of unconsciousness, fleeting periods of being asleep. But it's never proper sleep. It's fevered, brittle, pyretic – anything but restful. Often I'll get 'racing mind' – that phenomenon where the brain fixates on a tiny, often bizarre, topic for the whole night. I can't stop thinking about the ingredients for a recipe, or how to tie a tie, or the contents of my desk drawers. These inexplicable, odd thoughts whizz around my mind endlessly. And if I am lucky enough to drift off for a few minutes, I don't get proper dreams. They're only ever short, staccato ones; mini-episodes rather than the glorious feature films of proper slumber.

Insomnia is an anxiety disorder's wet dream because it's one of the few areas where the worries come true. Your thoughts can't stop your heart beating or prevent your lungs filling with air, but they *can* stop you sleeping. The more you think about sleep, the more you panic, and the less likely it is to happen. The prophecy becomes self-fulfilling.

Little wonder then that I've had tons – I mean *shit loads* – of sleepless nights since my breakdown. In fact, I had a 'non-starter' just last night. God, it was annoying. And completely random, too. I hadn't drunk coffee too late or stared at my phone too much. I can't even blame it on the upstairs neighbours (aka The Battersea Clog Dancing Team), who were abnormally quiet. It just came out of nowhere. 'I'm never going to sleep tonight' just popped into my head while I was brushing my teeth, and that was that.

The insomnia itself is maddening and saddening, but the days after it are worse. In our flat we call them Zombie Days. Although they're not really 'days' – they're expanses of time to be endured.

On a Zombie Day like today my whole body feels heavy, tender, cramped. My lower back feels taut and constricted, as though wrapped tightly in cling film. My hair, despite a shower, is flat and lank. My skin is bloated and blotchy. My nose is blocked. My sinuses throb. My eyes are itchy. My lips are dry. There's a dull headache at the front of my skull. I don't have an appetite. I'm cold.

Then there's the mental stuff. The phrase 'I'll never sleep again' has been whirring around my mind since morning. As has 'I'll never stop worrying about sleeping.' I've even had a bit of 'Maybe I'm going back to square one.' Ugh. Imagine that. Imagine going back to those first few weeks of pure panic after *that fucking party*. Imagine how long it would take to get better.

Of course I've been trying to do all the things that help. I've been trying to catch the thoughts and challenge them. I've tried concentrated breathing. I've done a guided meditation using an app on my phone. I've been to the gym. It's just harder to fight when you're knackered. I just want it to be over. Not *over*, over. I don't think today's a day for suicidal contemplation. I just want the thoughts to go away. I just want it to be tomorrow, today.

HIGH—FUNCTIONING ANXIOUS MAN

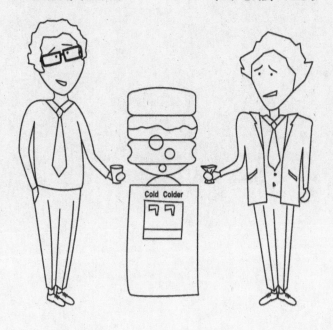

HIGH–FUNCTIONING ANXIOUS MAN

LIFE IS FULL of little surprises. Did you know, for example, that honey never goes off? Or that the capital of Nigeria *isn't* Lagos? Or that you can get free green tea in Wagamama? Or that people with anxiety disorders can seem entirely normal on the outside, while disintegrating on the inside?

It isn't the only surprise of my condition. For instance, I also had no idea just how physical mental health problems can be. When someone says that they feel nervous, they really do. They *feel* nervousness – in their heart rate, in their stomach, in the tightness of their skin and in their breath. And I hadn't a clue how prevalent anxiety disorders are. But this business of duality – the fact that I can seem outwardly fine while internally I am dying – is definitely the biggest surprise.

It truly is bizarre.

I can be at a dinner party, or in a meeting, or playing football, or writing, or shagging, and appear good. No, better

ANXIOUS MAN

than good. I can seem great. I can be on sparkling form. I can be 'Bloody great, thanks!', while at the same time imploding inside. It's as though I have two brains working separately, but simultaneously. One brain will be telling a joke in the pub, while the other will be saying 'You're never going to enjoy life because you'll always be worried about sleeping.'

Because of this duality, most of my friends had no idea how bad things were. It wasn't their fault, of course. How could they know? Having two brains meant that I still did all the stuff from before (squash, pub quizzes, watching the rugby, etc.), and I was largely the same as before, too. They had no way of knowing that I was crumbling; that, internally, my mind was only misery.

I suppose some of them noticed the lifestyle changes that came with the OCD – the not drinking, the exercise, the walking, for example. But a lot of that stuff was obscured by the general trend among my peers towards sobriety and 'cleaner' living. In the past 'I'm actually off booze at the moment' would have been met with extreme suspicion and derision. Nowadays no one bats an eyelid.

In a similar vein, I guess some friends would have clocked my needing to be busy. But, again, I don't think many of them would complain. After all, it's nice to be in demand. And I wasn't asking them to do anything weird, just to come along to the cinema or join me for an exercise class. My long-suffering best mate, Spence, is the only one who had to do something weird – a two-man trip paintballing. The less said about that the better.

Only a few people really knew the true state of things. My wonderful flatmate Adriana was one of them. She was the one who found me whispering 'I'm so fucked' on the kitchen floor. Poor Adriana. She really bore the brunt of it. For some reason (most likely because she's a babe), it just used to spill out of me. I talked to her endlessly about the trauma in my head, and crowbarred my thoughts into our interactions. Even the most simple, innocuous conversations would somehow come back to my anxiety.

'I was thinking fajitas for dinner,' she'd say.

'I don't know,' I'd reply. 'The last time we had fajitas I was really nervous the next day, and I've been feeling really down recently too.'

'Stir-fry it is then!'

It was different with Cali. I never deliberately hid it from my friends (it mostly hid itself), but with Cali I did. I actively concealed it from her, or tried to at least. My logic was simple: it was bad enough that I was trapped in an endless circle of anxiety, depression and obsessive compulsion; the last thing I wanted was for our relationship to suffer. I wanted to protect her – to protect *us* – from it. I wanted everything to seem fine, to be fine.

We did speak about it occasionally, but only ever loosely and euphemistically. My concern was that the contents of my head would freak her out. Or that my anxiety would take over our relationship. Or that she'd come to the conclusion that it'd all become too much like hard work. So I kept it vague, genteel and, well, quite British. 'Cripes I'm feeling a bit nervy today,' I'd say. Or 'Gosh I hope I sleep well tonight.'

Keeping schtum had the benefit of shielding our relationship from the day-to-day drama of my condition. But there was a downside, too. By not talking about it openly with Cali, I prevented her from gaining an understanding of what was going on. I was giving her enough information to worry (about me, about our relationship), but not enough to know what I was actually feeling. Like when your parents send you a 'please call me' text without any further explanation.

Eventually I realised the effects of the secrecy, and decided to go the other way. Too far the other way, actually. Very quickly my condition became a part of our dialogue, a big tenet of our relationship. I started dropping my anxious and intrusive thoughts into conversations or WhatsApp messages. They started to dominate our everyday lives.

'Penny for your thoughts,' she'd ask me on a long car journey.

'Not much really,' I'd say. 'Just thinking about driving the car onto the pavement.'

Quite understandably, the unfiltered honesty freaked her out and after two weeks we decided to have a conversation. What we agreed was that if I was desperate, or if the thoughts were really bad, we could talk about my anxiety. But that mostly it would be better to speak to a professional. We've kept it like this ever since, and it's worked a treat. We know where we stand. I know that I can talk to her if I need to, and she knows that she can send me to a professional if she wants to. Perfect.

Work was tricky. Not because the job itself was tricky – any human being (and most chimpanzees) could sell advertising to banks. Instead the challenge was trying to care. Or trying to *look* like I cared. The stuff in my head – the anxiety, the self-hatred, the compulsions – just seemed much more important than anything in my inbox. My thoughts were so severe, so existential, that work began to seem pointless. When you spend all day worrying about stabbing yourself in the neck or dying alone, it's really hard to get fired up about the latest sales push or the upgrade to Microsoft Office 365 (even if it does have tons of cool features).

Somehow, though, I mostly got away with it. I didn't miss any work because of my anxiety, and I don't think my colleagues clocked what was going on. Or perhaps they did, but didn't care. Either way, it didn't come up and I didn't really push it.

I've often wondered if I should have. I've questioned whether my silence at work makes me a bad mental health advocate. After all, how can we expect companies to get better at supporting people with problems if no one ever comes forward? But then again, everyone's entitled to a private life and, besides, I didn't *want* to talk about it. Boring as it was (and believe me it was *very* boring), work did at least provide some escape. It gave me things to think about that weren't worrisome, depressive or obsessive. Occasionally – very occasionally – it was absorbing enough to banish the anxiety entirely. And so the last thing I wanted to do was dredge up my misery through conversations with colleagues.

There were a few moments when the mask slipped, when my true state of mind burst through. One work trip in particular comes to mind.

I'd been sent to Geneva to cheer up some grumpy clients. I can't remember exactly why they were in a huff, but they were. In fact, they were so perturbed that at one point during the meeting I actually noticed some emotion creeping across their faces (this is an absolute 'no-no' for the Swiss).

The problem was that I just didn't care. Worse, I couldn't even muster the energy to pretend. 'What's the worst that can happen?' I remember thinking. 'What's the worst they can do?' Hit me with a cuckoo clock? Drown me in delicious milk chocolate ('made by Master Chocolatiers since 1845')? No, the worst that they could do would be to email my boss. That would be a bore – there'd have to be a 'catch-up coffee' and probably an apology note – but it would also be manageable. Once I realised that, I gave up caring completely. I surrendered to the apathy and spent the rest of the meeting staring out of the window, lusting after the lake, the hills, the mountains. You can say what you like about Switzerland (e.g. it's small, very expensive and full of tax-evading bores), but it is beautiful.

It took a week before the email arrived. 'They're saying you seemed distant,' my boss said. 'Is everything OK?'

I sat silently for a few seconds deciding what to say. I could come clean, I thought. I could tell him everything – how I'd been miserable for months, how I hadn't slept in weeks, how I kept worrying, and worrying about worrying, and how I hated myself. Maybe it would feel good to confess. Maybe it would lighten the load. Maybe it would make the anxiety go away. Yeah, fuck it. I'm going to confess, I said to myself. I'm going to do it. I'm going to tell the truth. I'm going to fucking do it. 'Well the truth is . . .' I said, pausing. 'The truth is . . . I'm completely fine.'

It has changed me, mind you. The breakdown, the anxiety, the obsession, the depression – it's changed me deeply and profoundly. I'm quieter these days, for example. And I'm more emotional. I cry more. My tears, once buried underneath six feet of masculine bravado, are now barely concealed. It used to take a 'military vet reunited with pet' video to set me off. Now just seeing Cali at the end of a long day is enough. Plus my temper is shorter. Refracted through my worried brain, life's small irritations take on much bigger significance. A stubbed toe becomes a reason to throw something; a parking fine leads to a punched wall.

But, despite all of this, I have survived. My condition hasn't been a death sentence. Having an anxiety disorder hasn't been the end.

It's been infuriating, exhausting and frightening, as well as a catastrophic waste of life (every day spent anxious is a day *not spent* laughing, learning, experiencing the world). But it's also been manageable and 'get-better-able'.

WHY ME?

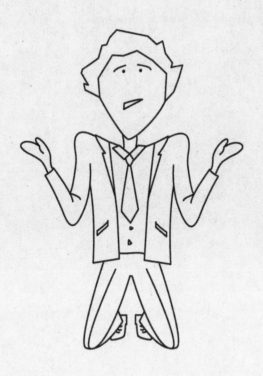

WHY ME?

THERE ARE TWO main theories about the causes of mental health problems. For simplicity, I'll call them 'the parents one' and 'the environment one'.

The parents one is fairly self-explanatory. It's the idea that mental health problems, like many physical ones, are passed down through families. Genetics is the obvious mechanism; mental ill health could be preprogrammed into our DNA from birth. Or parents could pass it on by exhibiting depressive or anxious behaviours themselves. As children we learn everything from observing and copying our parents – including, potentially, how to be depressed or anxious.

In contrast, the environment one suggests that it's all about individuals, their behaviour and the things that happen in their lives. Everyone has the propensity to worry or be depressed, and it's what happens/how people behave that determines if they will. Drinking too much alcohol, taking drugs and not sleeping enough could all be causes. As could getting fired, being dumped or losing someone.

So which one is it? Well, sadly, nobody's sure. Despite lots of effort and money, the science isn't yet conclusive. It's not the boffins' fault; it's just extremely difficult to research mental health. Not only because the brain is so wonderfully complex, but also it's really difficult to design robust trials.

With physical health it's easier, as you can determine the role of genetics by conducting trials on sets of twins. This doesn't work with mental health, however, because you can't control for all the variables. If, for example, both twins develop depression, it could be because they have the same 'depressive genes' or it could be because they've both had rotten lives. One could have been laid off work, while the other might have been abused as a child.

The research is also plagued with logical challenges. For example, lots of research shows that people with depression have smaller hippocampi (the hippocampus is the area of the brain involved in memory-forming). But that only proves correlation, not causation. Does a smaller hippocampus cause depression, or does depression result in a smaller hippocampus? It's a chicken-and-egg kinda thing.

In my own case, I think it was a bit of both. Depression and anxiety hang off my family tree like miserable black blossom. And I reckon that, plus things like societal pressures and the way I behaved through my twenties (more on both of these later), was what tipped me over the edge.

I didn't always think like this. When I first broke down I was convinced that it was all down to me and my reckless behaviour, and not just due to the circumstances of my breakdown (the morning after *that fucking party*). I also *wanted* that to be the case. Because if it was, then it would be easier to fix. If it was all down to bad behaviour, then all I had to do was behave better, and the anxiety would evaporate. The alternative – having a genetic problem – would be much harder, if not impossible, to fix.

It took a year before I accepted that other factors could be involved. Over that time it just became obvious. On two different days I'd behave exactly the same (not drink, exercise, etc.) and yet experience wildly differing levels of anxiety. Clearly something else was going on. It could be genetics, or it could be complete randomness. Either way, it wasn't all me.

Realising this was scary. As a species, we humans crave certainty. We hate risk. We despise 'not knowing'. Everything must have an explanation. Everything must happen for a reason. Whenever we can't explain something we go to pieces. 'Not knowing' makes us do weird things like buy insurance, visit clairvoyants and invent religions.

I'm no exception to this. Accepting the randomness and uncertainty of my condition was terrifying because it also meant accepting that there was nothing I could do about it. If nothing specific causes it, then nothing specific can prevent it. I could change jobs, go teetotal and exercise loads and still be anxious. It would just happen, like traffic jams or Easter. But there were also two distinct upsides to this realisation.

The first was that it allowed me to end my mad quest for a cause. And with that, I began to unpick all the bizarre rules, rituals and compulsions that had taken over my life. If there was no way of stopping my anxiety or depression, then there was no point going to bed at certain times, drinking certain amounts of water, walking a certain number of steps a day, and so on.

The other benefit was that I could stop hating myself. In the beginning I'd wanted my condition to be my fault because that would make it easier to fix. But as an unwanted byproduct I began to despise myself for it. I was to blame – I'd given myself the condition – and therefore I was a terrible person. If only I hadn't gone to that party. If only I'd been stronger and more resilient. If only I was normal. If only I wasn't so useless. *Why am I so fucking useless?*

It turns out that thoughts like these are extremely common. Everyone I've spoken to has not only blamed themselves for their condition, but also hated themselves for it. Maybe they could have done things differently, or not done certain things, or spotted the problem sooner. Perhaps they drank too much or took too many drugs. 'I just wish I could go back in time' is a common sentiment. As is 'If only I hadn't . . .'

Self-hatred like this is both grim and unhelpful. It's a distraction. It's just another thing that I have to unpick before I can get to the real problem underneath. Thankfully, though, it's also optional. I have to choose to blame and hate myself, and these days I don't bother. These days I don't care about what causes my anxiety, depression and obsession. Instead I focus on what really matters: getting better.

THE SHAME GAME

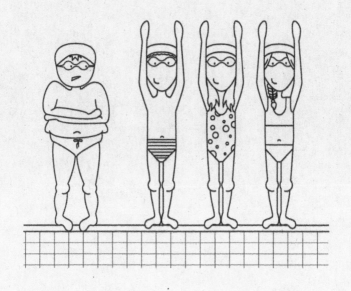

THE SHAME GAME

SOCIETAL EXPECTATIONS ARE funny old things.

I suppose some of them are quite handy. Without them – without some accepted behavioural norms – many of us would be a bit lost. We wouldn't know how to behave, what to say or how to form an orderly queue. In that sense, they're a kind of social glue binding together the human experience.

But societal expectations can also be bloody annoying things. No, worse – they can be terribly harmful. Because whenever we set expectations, we open up the possibility of missing those expectations. We create the potential for 'should'-style worries on a national scale. And that's incredibly dangerous.

For evidence of why, just look at Japan, which, since the eighties, has been in the grips of a terrifying suicide epidemic. There are lots of drivers behind the Japanese problem, but primarily it's a crisis born of societal expectations. Because in Japan, unlike almost anywhere else on earth, killing yourself can be the *right* thing to do. It's even accounted for in some

Japanese life insurance contracts. The thinking goes that if you can't provide for your family in life, you should do so by killing yourself. The fact that suicide rates spike in March (the end of the Japanese tax year) shows this grim duty in action.

But if the culture of suicide is different in the West, the idea of societal expectations is the same. We still set ludicrous, unachievable goals for one another. We still expect everyone to be thin, and successful, and happy; we just don't encourage suicide as an emergency exit. Our penalty for failure is more subtle, but no less pernicious. It's a cruel, living punishment called 'shame'.

The concept of shame is as old as humanity itself. Ever since we've had consciousness, we've been using it to create expectations for each other, and to goad each other when we fail. That said, the arbiters of social expectation have changed greatly throughout history. At the start they were religious; popes, priests, imams and bhikkhus were the ones deciding how society should think, look and behave, and they were the ones doling out punishments for failure. These were the days of pillories, public whippings, tarrings and featherings, head shavings, etc.

Thankfully, judicial corporal punishment was abolished in the UK in 1948. And that, combined with the explosion of cheap printing and the transition towards secularism, led to a change in public shaming personnel. More specifically, it resulted in newspaper and magazine editors assuming the role of Shamers in Chief.

Now it was they who decided what we should look like and how we should behave. And whenever someone failed to meet their rules, or dared to live outside of them, the deviants were splashed across the front pages with shrieking, exposing headlines. Celebrities were the natural targets. No one cares how celebs feel, and there's an almost endless supply of them. So, if someone put on weight, or made a bad career choice, or was addicted to alcohol, or dared to be a mother *and* have a career, the newspapers arrested them, exhibited them and shamed them.

But if the public shaming of the past was intense (and often hypocritical), it was at least contained. Through careful curation of your media intake you could mostly avoid it. If you didn't want to laugh along at the silly celebrities with depression, or dead parents, or disabled children, you didn't have to. Then social media happened.

Social media has revolutionised the way we shame. Not only has it created new, even more unattainable expectations of us and our lives, it's also equipped a new army of keyboard warriors with the means to judge, scream and shame. In the past we, the public, were largely passive participants. Now, we lead the charge. And it's not just celebrities that we focus on; now we like to do it to each other too. 'He's put on weight,' we say. 'Her wedding looked cheap', 'Why is she going out with him?', 'Shouldn't she be at home?', 'Their baby is ugly' . . .

My personal experience of shame started young. I was an obese child. Not a little bit fat, or a smidge overweight, but full-on obese. Indeed, for most of my childhood I had the body mass index of a prize-winning bluefin tuna. There were even moments when my weight in stone eclipsed my years in age. I was *that* big.

For a good few years it didn't bother me. Or at least it didn't enter my consciousness. I was fat, others weren't. Who cared? Then one day, aged eight, my attitude changed. I can vividly remember the exact moment that it happened.

At my primary school – a happy little place in Woking – we got two breaks in the morning. First break was all about hanging around in the playground trading Pokémon cards, throwing diabolos and exchanging *GoldenEye* tactics. It was cool, but it wasn't nearly as cool as second break. For at second break we got given a snack. Sometimes it was a doughnut, sometimes it was a Wagon Wheel or an Orange Club or a mini packet of Jammie Dodgers. On the day in question, however, it was none of those things. Instead it was my favourite snack, the Best Snack in the World: hot, crunchy, buttered toast smothered with a thick slick of Nutella. It was the sole reason for going to school on Mondays. It was everything. And so as soon as the bell rang on this particular day, I packed up my pencil case, legged it to the dining room, pushed past the queue, ducked around the prefect checking for clean hands, squeezed through the door and charged towards the Formica table laden with toast.

Once there I gorged, gobbled, scoffed and stuffed. I chomped, and swallowed, and chomped some more. I munched with the frenzied ferocity of a starved piranha shoal. Crumbs filled the air. One slice of toast disappeared, then two, then three. I was lost in time, taken away by the buttery, hazelnutty hedonism of the moment – sheer, ecstatic, leg-shaking, gustatory climax.

I ate six slices of toast that day.

That wasn't my best performance (I'd managed eight a few weeks prior); an average performance, on an average day. What wasn't average, however, was the sensation that it left me with. Usually gobbling toast satisfied me, it made me happy. On this day – and I've no idea why – it made me feel embarrassed. Up until that point, I'd always worn my appetite and consumption with pride.

'How many slices did you manage?' my mate Chaz would ask on the way back to lessons.

'Six,' I'd reply triumphantly.

On that day, though, the only thing I felt was embarrassed. It was like I'd woken up to my greed and appearance. I felt hideous, gross and grotesque. Worse, for the first time, I felt abnormal. From that moment onwards I felt a deep shame about my appearance, and it stayed that way for years.

I despised being fat. I loathed my body. I hated the way it looked, the fact that I had bigger boobs than most of the girls at primary school. It was bad enough when clothed, and unbearable when not.

Take swimming lessons. Good lord I hated swimming lessons. I used to pray for a verruca so that I wouldn't have to go. It was as though the whole thing had been set up to ensure maximum embarrassment for me and the other fatty (a nice bloke called Tom). The outfits were the first humiliation. God knows why, but for some reason the school was very prescriptive when it came to swimwear. Shorts and trunks were outlawed; only Speedos were permitted. For the 'normal' kids I'm sure that was fine. For me, the ignominy was abject. Each week I had to squeeze my way into the damn things. Everyone else could get changed in a flash. Not me. I took 10 minutes to get ready – tugging, wrenching, hoicking at the dark blue Lycra until the Speedos were on.

Not that they were ever properly 'on'. They don't make Speedos to fit eight-stone eight-year-olds, so I had to be content with only partial corporal coverage. If I could get them to cover 50 per cent of my pink, blubbery bum then that would be a win.

Then there were the lessons themselves. The diving ones were the worst. At least if we were practising backstroke, or collecting a brick from the deep end, I could conceal myself under the water. With diving lessons that wasn't an option. I was forever standing on the side of the pool, exposed to the chilly June weather and to the sniggering stares of my classmates.

'Line up boys,' the swimming coach (a greasy bloke called Derek) would say. 'Alphabetical order please.'

Obediently, we'd shuffle into position along the edge of the outdoor, unheated swimming pool.

'When I say your name you will perform a dive into the pool and swim to the side,' said Derek. 'Anderson, go. Andrews, go. Bell, go. Cummings, go.'

I'd stand there shivering, wanting nothing more than to hear my name. 'If only I was Anderson's twin brother,' I'd say to myself. 'Then I could jump in now and hide my disgusting body.'

Then, after the lessons, came the indignity and horror of the changing room. It was a square, breeze-block thing that had been tacked on hurriedly at the end of the eighties. It was damp, musty and fetid. And that was before you added 200 pubescent boys in their dirty sports kit. Lockers – wire mesh ones – lined the four walls, meaning that we all got changed facing towards one another. And this dearth of privacy or personal space extended into the showers. Or, rather, into the single communal shower. Which, for some inexplicable reason, was supervised by the Religious Studies teacher. You wouldn't get away with that these days.

'You seem to have dropped your towel,' he'd say to his favourites. 'Better bend over and pick it up.'

Embarrassment, guilt and shame about my body followed me around outside of school, too. Clothes shopping, for example, was the pits. In the nineties, trying to clothe a portly child was an insuperable challenge. No one made clothes for kids with lumpen, short, fat frames like mine. And when we did chance upon something like an XXL T-shirt, or a pair of elasticated trousers, it was never from a cool brand that my friends wore. In fact, it was only ever from one shop: GAP. Actually, it was only ever one outfit: tracksuit bottoms, white T-shirt and a fleece that was blue on the bottom and grey on the top. I wore that same get-up every day for five years, like a tweenage Steve Jobs. Entire fashions and trends came and went – the surfer phase, the goth phase, the skater phase – and still my apparel remained steadfastly unchanged.

Holidays as a fatso were also fraught with embarrassment. Just like swimming lessons, you have to take off your top on holiday. I couldn't do that. I couldn't foist my big, flushed, wobbly torso on the other unsuspecting holidaymakers. Even getting it out in front of my family triggered angst. So instead I kept my T-shirt on at all times. Swimming, snorkelling, boogie boarding – it didn't matter. Whatever I was doing, I was doing it with my T-shirt on. I used to return from holidays with forearms browner than mahogany, but a chest whiter than Donald Trump's electoral base.

By the age of nine I was such a porker that a trip to the dietician became inevitable. A routine visit to the GP resulted in a referral, and within a week I found myself sitting in front of Miss Merriweather. She was a kind-looking lady, probably about the same age as I am now, who nodded quietly and reassuringly as my mum read out my weekly food diary.

'On Saturday his snacks were an apple in the morning and Soreen malt loaf in the afternoon,' said my mum.

'OK, that's not too bad,' said Miss Merriweather. 'How many slices of Soreen malt loaf exactly?'

'Erm,' said Mum, considering a lie. 'Actually he had a whole one.' A pause. 'Buttered.'

That was the beginning of the end for fat me. Overnight, my portions at home became radically smaller. While at school my eating habits began to be scrutinised by the teachers. Even my old allies, the dinner ladies, were in on the betrayal.

'Please, Brenda, may I have an extra turkey twizzler?' I remember asking.

'Sorry, wee Josh,' she said in her lilting Scottish burr. 'Canne do it. Headmaster says so. Only normal portions from now on.' Et tu, Brenda?

The upside of dieting, of course, was that the weight began to melt away. By the time I went to boarding school, aged 13, it had nearly normalised completely. And, aside from the indulgence of university, it's stayed that way ever since.

There are lots of complicated reasons why people overeat. For some it's a form of self-harm, for others it's a self-reinforcing, cyclical sort of thing. As Fat Bastard so eloquently put it in *Austin Powers*: 'I eat because I'm unhappy, and I'm unhappy because I eat.'

For me, though, the motivation for gorging and munching was much simpler: I just liked eating delicious things. I still do. I'm still greedy. I'm still a glutton. I'm still powerless in front of buttery, sweet popcorn and deliciously dark chocolate. I still crumble for crumble, pine for pasta, yearn for Yorkie bars. The difference is that these days I'm able to exercise a degree of self-control. It's by no means total. From time to time my rapacity for saturated fats and simple carbohydrates takes over. But mostly I can keep myself on the straight and narrow. Case in point: I'm writing this in May and I still haven't finished my Easter egg. To a pre-teen me this would have seemed psychopathic. To Cali, it still does.

Bedtime was my other source of childhood shame. For the entirety of my youth I was completely terrified of the dark. Or, more accurately, I was completely terrified of being murdered in the dark. I have no idea why or where this fear came from. It hadn't happened before – we hadn't even been burgled. And yet, for years, I was totally convinced that a

73

masked assailant was going to break into the house and start murdering us all.

I thought about it every night. After brushing my teeth, I'd climb into my bed, pull my Manchester United duvet cover over and imagine the sequence of events that was about to unfold. I imagined seeing my bedroom door open, watching as the assailant approached my bed, glimpsing the large knife in his right hand, trying to scream, feeling the cold steel against my throat, the warm trickle of blood, the choking, the darkness.

It was like that each night of the week. Usually I'd spend a couple of hours worrying before eventually trundling along to my parents' room. At first they let me climb into their bed; and when that became impractical (due to my ever-expanding dimensions) they kindly put a camp bed in the corner. I slept there every night for five years.

In the end, just like with my weight, it got bad enough that specialist help became unavoidable.

Mrs Stephenson was a 60-year-old spinster with a wispy white moustache and breath that smelled of Marmite. She called herself a paediatric sleep therapist, but her 'clinic' was so informal that, even aged 10, I had my doubts about her credibility.

Sessions took place in the conservatory of her semi-detached home in West Byfleet. There was a comfy chair, a glass of Ribena and a CD of whale music. Mrs Stephenson would have me sit in the chair and close my eyes before pressing play on the whale music. Then she'd begin mumbling on about warm, cosy, safe places and instruct me to think certain things.

Invariably, and unsurprisingly given how knackered I was, I'd drift off to sleep within 10 minutes and stay that way until the end of the hour-long, £60 appointment. Nice little business that: £60 to watch a kid sleep for 55 minutes. Although I doubt she did actually watch me – I'm convinced that she had different children asleep in different rooms.

Needless to say, Mrs Stephenson's 'therapy' had no impact whatsoever. It wasn't until I went to boarding school that I got better at sleeping. Being scared of the dark wasn't really an option there. I had no choice but to get over it. Although I've never got over it completely. I still hate being in the house on my own. I still prefer to sleep with the bedroom door locked. Adriana busted me doing it once. 'You do realise that I hear you locking your door at night,' she said one morning.

It happened, by the way. My premonition about waking up to find an intruder in the house came true. It was on holiday in Greece a few years ago. Thankfully, he didn't steal much and I didn't get murdered (as you can tell). In fact, the reality was nothing like I'd imagined for all those years. Oddly, it wasn't as scary. I just woke up to find a man rustling through the bedside table. I shouted at him and he legged it. I even gave chase. Which was a weird choice given (a) the size of the bloke and (b) the fact that I was sleeping naked (I come over all European on hot holidays). To this day I don't know if it was my shouting or the sight of my sunburned birthday suit that scared him more.

I've often wondered whether the shame I felt in my child-hood is a cause or symptom of my current condition. Do I worry now *because* of it? Or is it just further evidence that I've always been a worrier?

I'm not sure either way, but I do think that I learned shame at a young age, and that I've carried that capability into adulthood. The way I reacted to my mental health diagnosis is a perfect example.

I mentioned earlier that I felt a weird blend of relief and fear at being diagnosed with an anxiety disorder, and I did. But my primary emotion sitting in the doctor's surgery was shame. Partly it was about being weak. But also because, well, I should be happy. I'm a white, middle-class, heterosexual man for goodness sake. It's not possible to imagine a life less worrisome than mine. I've never been oppressed or discriminated against. I've never been abused or neglected, or lonely. I've never had to struggle. *What on earth do I have to worry about?*

The answer, obviously, is nothing. I don't have anything to worry about. I just happen to have a condition that makes me do it. It's a condition that anyone can develop. It's a condition that doesn't care if I'm rich or poor, male or female, black or white, gay or straight. Just as I shouldn't feel guilty for having multiple sclerosis, I shouldn't feel shame for having depression or anxiety.

It took me two years to realise this. It was a conversation with a therapist that did it.

'Why don't you like discussing your problems?' he asked.

'Because it's embarrassing,' I said. 'I hate the idea of being just another privileged bloke with a mental health problem.'

'I do hope you'll excuse my French,' came his response, 'but that is complete bullshit. The only reason you think this is a middle-class problem is because the middle classes are the ones who can get help. You've got a universal problem, and I suggest we start fixing it.'

So we did.

MAN UP, BREAK DOWN

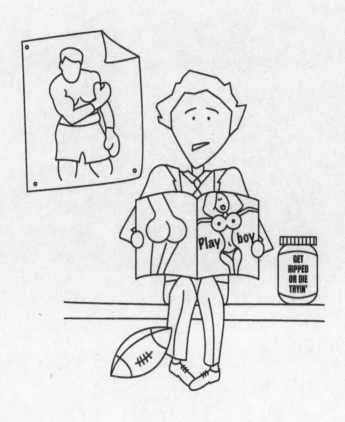

MAN UP, BREAK DOWN

DESPITE MY WEIGHT and sleeping issues, for the most part I was a happy boy. A happy boy, in a happy family.

There are five of us in my family – me, my two older brothers (Tom and Ben), and my mum and dad. Dad worked in technology. Mum gave up a career designing interiors to look after me and my brothers. Our house, a pretty Tudor one on the outskirts of a quiet village, was one filled with laughter and love.

Materially, too, we were pretty comfortable. We weren't allowed fizzy drinks, oven chips or Sky TV, but I did have a Micro scooter, a Tamagotchi and a Nerf gun. Weekends were always packed with fun activities like sailing, bike rides and bonfires. And Sunday lunch was a big deal. Some folks hesitate when you ask them what their death row meal would be. I don't. I know exactly what I'd order. I'd want any of the Sunday roasts from my childhood: roast chicken cooked by my mother, apple crumble and a lively family debate about the merits of getting a go-kart. Followed, of course, by a postprandial episode of *Scrapheap Challenge*.

For a family that is 80 per cent men, I'd say that our home was surprisingly unmasculine. It wasn't feminine either; it just wasn't masculine. None of us supported football teams, or shouted at the rugby, or did that golf thing. I guess there were quite a few copies of *Classic Cars* magazine in the downstairs loo, but that's about as 'geezery' as we got.

These days I do a bit more of the conventional 'man' stuff. I'm not averse to a stag do, for example. And I love DIY. Last year I even bought a season ticket for Fulham FC – up the Whites! (NB this is a reference to Fulham's white kit, and not a racial slur) – but I gave it up after one season. It was just too boring.

Given how un-blokey I feel, it's surprising how much traditional ideals of masculinity have affected my life. I've moved house when I didn't want to, taken jobs I didn't want, slept with girls I didn't like, and dumped one that I did – all because I wanted to be a 'good lad'. Which is bizarre, not least because what constitutes a 'good lad' is so nebulous.

Ten years ago it was more straightforward. Back then, us chaps knew where we stood. We knew that we were supposed to like football, drink beer, eat curries (spicy ones only) and fancy women. And we knew that we should listen to Oasis, read *Nuts* magazine and watch Men & Motors. Sadly, we weren't allowed to engage with our feelings or emotions. And books, too, were outlawed. Unless we were holidaying with 'a bird', in which case a copy of *Bravo Two Zero* or *The World According to Clarkson* might be permitted. But even that was pushing it. Caring about our appearance was also strictly prohibited. Mostly we wore supermarket denim and rugby shirts. Unless we were 'going out on the pull', in which case it was ill-fitting jeans, an untucked (100 per cent polyester) black shirt and pointy tan loafers. And as for grooming, hair gel and a blob of 'the missus's moisturiser' was OK, but anything else was asking for trouble.

The 'lad culture' definition of masculinity was both ludicrous and harmful, but it was at least settled. Most of us didn't identify with it, and lots of us felt uncomfortable with it, but we did at least know what 'it' was. These days, that isn't always the case. Over the past 10 years, what it means to be a man has changed rapidly and irrevocably. And society's expectations of men have shifted, too. In general, we're still expected to be rock solid, James Bond badasses. It's just that we're also supposed to do a bunch of other stuff as well.

ADVERT

Modern society seeks modern man for love, laughter and confusing, unattainable standards of masculinity. The perfect man will be:

- Tall (but not too tall)
- Handsome (but in an unknowing way)
- Toned (without trying too hard)
- Feminist (without virtue signalling)
- Hard-working (again, just not too much)
- Funny (without being showy-offy)
- Hard (in all senses)
- Provider (but never patronising)
- Vulnerable (just without compromising any of the above)

In the long term, the transition towards a broader, more fluid and more welcoming masculinity will be hugely positive – for men, women and everyone else. But there's also a risk that the new requirements of manhood add to, rather than replace, the old ones. Which is dangerous because it could mean even more unattainable expectations, and even more men feeling not enough. And make no mistake, lots of blokes don't feel enough. Why else would suicide be the biggest killer of men under the age of 50?

The answer, of course, is for us to talk about it. To talk about how we really feel, what we really think and what we really want. Sadly, we've never been much good at that. Particularly when it comes to mental health. It isn't really our fault. Up until relatively recently, science didn't consider it possible for men to develop mental health problems. Given that hysteria and melancholia (ye olde anxiety and depression) were 'caused' by movements in the uterus, men couldn't develop them. And as a result, we couldn't talk about them. After all, you can't admit to a problem that you can't have.

Like many men, I wasn't really aware of mental health growing up. It never came up. It wasn't part of my world. None of my friends or teachers had experienced problems. And even though, looking back, I can see evidence of mental health issues in my family, it wasn't like we discussed them around the kitchen table. We did have one family friend who took an 'emergency sabbatical'. But even that was explained away with a 'he's been working too hard'. Nowadays we'd call that 'burnout' – a clever linguistic compromise that allows blokes to admit weakness, while maintaining their machismo ('I work so fucking hard, because I'm such a fucking **man**, that I literally fucking *burned out*').

Because male mental health isn't really talked about, when we do have mental health problems, we rarely ask for help. And because we don't ask for help, our problems just get worse and worse, until eventually we decide that we can't do it any longer. So we find a rope, or go to the train station and just get it over with.

That's what happened with my mate Max who had the car crash on the M1. And my pal Pete. He's an army man. Or at least he was. He left at the end of last year, having missed a promotion. That's how it started – his anxiety, depression and feeling 'not enough'. It didn't help that he'd just become a father: 'How am I supposed to provide if I can't even get a fucking promotion?'

It only took three months for Pete to attempt suicide. He did it with an overdose. Or at least, he tried to. Thankfully, I think given his size, it didn't work. His wife found him slumped on the sofa, and now he's getting better. I had lunch with him recently.

'I've been doing that therapy shite,' he said. 'I'm going absolutely fuckin' mad fer it.'

I should have said – Pete's from Manchester.

It wasn't until my twenties – and Max's car crash – that I first properly encountered male mental illness. And even then, I'll admit that I was sceptical. I might even have written it off as 'attention-seeking'. I wouldn't dream of doing that now. Now that I know how real mental ill health is. Now that

I know the pain in breaking, and being broken. Now that I know the effort, exhaustion and agony of recovery.

There were two reasons why I kept quiet about my anxiety disorder at work.

The first, I mentioned earlier – work provided a partial escape from my thoughts, and I wanted to preserve that. The second reason, though, was more troubling. I didn't confess to having a problem, because I was scared to. It's hard to write that, but it's true. I was frightened about what my colleagues, especially the male ones, would think of me. I thought that admitting to being broken would mark me out as a problem child. I thought that the bosses would write me off. I thought that it would fuck up my career. I thought that having a weakness, being broken, *feeling* was incompatible with being a successful man.

Eventually, however, I had to come clean. It just became inevitable. I simply couldn't hide the unhappiness, disinterest and crying in the bogs any longer. So I booked meetings with my boss, my boss's boss and the big boss (all of them blokes), and confessed.

What happened next was both surprising and brilliant. Not only did all three of them offer empathy and support, but two of them had actually had similar problems themselves. And these aren't what you'd consider modern, metropolitan men. These are veterans of advertising sales – one of the most alpha-male industries imaginable.

The experience taught me two things. Firstly, that, on the whole, humans are great. And, secondly, that mental health problems are much, much more prevalent than I thought. In fact, 25 per cent of people will experience one in their lifetime. Which means that, assuming most people have three friends, 100 per cent of the population will either have a problem themselves or know someone who has. In other words, when you confess to depression or anxiety, you'll likely be pushing on an open door.

If there's one thing you remember from this, I'd like it to be that. Because the sooner we admit to a problem, the sooner we get help. Mental health problems are cancers of the mind – catch them early and recovery is possible, there is hope; but leave them alone and they grow much bigger and much harder to remove. Early intervention is key.

WORLDWIDE WORRY

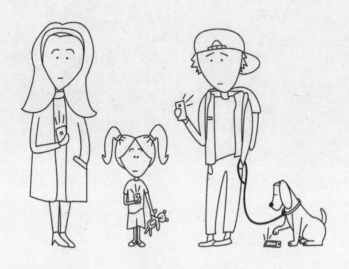

WORLDWIDE WORRY

WORLDWIDE WORRY

AS SOMEONE BORN in 1990, I'm quite well placed to assess the impacts of social media. I'm old enough to remember a life before 'likes' and 'shares', but young enough to know how it all works, and to have got stuck in.

For me, it all began with Bebo. Myspace was cooler and older than Bebo, but it was also populated by trendy day school kids and I found its focus on music overwhelming. Don't get me wrong, I love music. It's just my musical tastes are what Cali describes as 'objectively shit'. Plus I've never been good at remembering bands. I recall once being asked to name my favourite rapper. 'Erm,' I paused, trying to think of *any* rapper. 'Shaggy?'

The other thing I liked about Bebo was its clarity. It was a pure, unadulterated popularity contest. Sure, you could post pictures of each other, and you could comment on each other's pages, but that was only ever a sideshow – the 'media' entrée to the 'social' main course. It was a popularity pageant and everyone knew it.

There were a few ways that you could tell someone's popularity on Bebo. Their number of friends, obviously. As well as the 'view counter' handily displayed underneath their profile picture – more views, more popular, obvs. But by far the most brutal way of measuring popularity was a feature called the 'Top 10' – a little corner of your profile page where you listed your top 10 best mates. Although in reality it was much more complicated and much, much more political than that.

I was a peripheral member of my school's cool gang. I don't think I was a total loser, but I definitely wasn't a bona fide insider. I usually needed a good reason to sit with them at lunch, and I had to graft for party invites and group holidays. All of which I was fine with. I don't think I could have handled being a proper cool-ganger anyway – too much swearing at teachers, not nearly enough Debating Soc.

The downside of being on the edges of coolness, however, was that I was particularly vulnerable to the changing winds of the Bebo 'Top 10s'. Snog the wrong girl, or wear the wrong trainers, and I could find myself exiled to social Siberia; disappeared from 'Top 10s' like a North Korean dissident. I know this because it actually happened. Ugh, I'll never forget it – the day Myles got caught smoking weed.

I don't remember the month exactly, but it was definitely the summer term – that weird bit in between exams finishing and the holidays starting. Everyone was just sat about waiting, yearning for the summer to arrive. And it was in this febrile environment that Myles got caught.

To understand how seismically cool it was to get caught smoking 'ganja', you have to remember that I was at a very strict boarding school. We weren't allowed chewing gum, or dyed hair, or even mobile phones. So to get busted *smoking an actual spliff* was incredible. It was just the most earth-shatteringly, pant-wettingly rebellious and epic thing ever.

Immediately, people began tripping over themselves to include Myles in their Bebo Top 10. Which was good news for Myles, but terrible news for the socially vulnerable (aka me). In just a few hours I went from being in six Top 10s, to being in none. From contented peripheral, to social pariah in an afternoon. It took me at least a term to recover socially. Psychologically, I'm not sure I ever will.

Like most teen obsessions, our fascination with Bebo didn't last long. In 2006 Facebook arrived, and with that everything changed. The initial allure of Facebook was its age restriction. At the start you had to be at university to open an account, and aged 16 we thought that was awesome. But if that's what drew us in, what made us engage and obsess over Facebook was the product itself. It was just better than Bebo. It allowed us to connect with people in new, exciting ways. We could privately message people we didn't know. We could create group chats. We could organise events. We could 'poke' people. We could even spend hours and hours sneakily stalking our exes. It became a conversation starter, a conversation dominator. It became the centre of the social world. And, for the first time, that social world was available 24/7/365.

Bebo whet our whistles, but it was Facebook that really taught us how to 'do' social media. It was the cool cousin showing us how to smoke, the older girlfriend guiding us through sex. It taught us how to fake our lives, how to obsess over others' and how to be angry. It wasn't long before other platforms sprang up to service those needs more specifically. Instagram, for example, has largely captured the 'how to fake our lives, and obsess over others'' bit. And if it's anger you're after, Twitter is the one for you.

I've been properly addicted to social media for five years. And, for the avoidance of doubt, addiction is absolutely the right word. It's the first thing I do in the morning, and the last thing I do at night. I do it wherever I am in the world, and whatever I happen to be doing. I do it while watching television, while chatting with friends, while sitting on the loo. Whenever there's a small break in my day, my hand – guided by a Pavlovian muscle memory – reaches into my pocket, unlocks the screen, opens an app (usually Instagram) and begins scrolling. In the past week alone, I opened my phone 242 times a day, and spent over nine hours cruising social media.

The only thing I can liken it to is smoking cigarettes (I used to be a 20-a-day man). The parallels between the two are uncanny. Just as with lighting my first cigarette, for example, I tend to check my social feeds within 10 minutes of waking up. And I look forward to it in the same way I used to with fags. As soon as the meeting ends, the train arrives or the plane lands, I'm straight onto it.

I also fabricate stories and circumstances to let me consume it. I used to do this with cigarettes the whole time. 'Just popping to the shops,' I'd say. Or 'I don't mind walking the dog.' When really all I wanted to do was smoke a ciggie. With social media it's a bit more subtle, but no less contrived. 'Have you seen the pics of Jamie's holiday?' I'll say while, without waiting for an answer, getting my phone out. Or 'Can I show you this video?'

Probably the saddest similarity between 'social' and ciggies is that I need it. I think that a scroll of Twitter, or a peruse of Instagram, improves my day. It was the same with smoking. I thought that a quick Marlboro Light made my day better than other people's. I thought cigarettes elevated my existence above the norm. In reality, the opposite was true (I needed nicotine to enjoy the peace and contentment that non-smokers get for free), but I didn't think that at the time.

Which brings me to the final, most important parallel between smoking fags and using social media: I know that it's bad for me, and yet I continue to do it. I know that it mostly makes me unhappy, angry and anxious, but still I scroll, and scroll, and scroll. Still I hook myself up to an intravenous drip of vapid, vacuous bullshit of the sort that arseholes call 'content'.

The research into social media and mental health is worrying, if unsurprising. Almost all the studies suggest that the more time someone spends on social, the more likely they are to suffer depression and anxiety. Young people are particularly susceptible – the explosion of social media has coincided with a 50 per cent increase in childhood mental health problems.

In my own case, I'd stop short of saying that social media caused my condition, but it certainly hasn't made it any better. Why would it? Why would consuming curated, if not entirely invented, versions of other people's lives make me feel better about my own?

And, by the way, they really are invented. Most social media is complete fiction. All those big smiles, fun-looking parties, expensive-looking holidays – they're all made up. Or at the very least, they're constructed to seem bigger, more fun and more expensive than they really are.

I suspect you know all this, but I also suspect that you don't care. I reckon you know that those lithe bodies and chiselled faces are fake, but that you crack on and compare yourself to them anyway. That's what I used to do. I used to spend hours gawking at 'influencers' (eurgh) driving free Lamborghinis and cursing myself for not being able to buy one.

I've used the past tense there, because these days I try not to do all that. I still go on social media (loads). I just only follow cheery things or things that interest me – fancy architecture, funny pets, that sort of stuff. Which I don't mean in a virtue signalling, 'aren't I so wholesome and countercultural' kind of way. I just had a moment last year when the ersatz boasting, bullshitting and fakery of social media was made so plain to me that I decided to switch it up.

My friend Liz had been unceremoniously dumped by her boyfriend of three years by text (I know, what a knob), and I'd taken her for a pizza to commiserate. The poor thing just cried, and cried, and cried. Hot tears falling on her American Hot. She didn't even touch the dough balls. It was heartbreaking to see her so upset, and to see so much good dough go to waste. Worst of all, there was nothing that I could do to help. It was desperate and I left the restaurant feeling mortified for her. Then, later that evening, I checked my Instagram and my sadness turned to bafflement. 'SUCH a great evening,' read Liz's latest post accompanying a smiley selfie. 'You can't beat Pizza Express.'

'How would you know?' I remember thinking. 'You only had one slice.'

After that I gave up caring about 'social'. Who wouldn't? If it's all fabricated, if the whole thing is one giant game of 'opposites day', if its sole purpose is to construct and project wildly untrue, outlandishly aspirational pretend lives, then, well, what's the fucking point?

Have you ever been watching television when they've cut unexpectedly to the news? It's happened to me twice. Once after the 2005 London bombings, and again after Mandela died. Both times I found it electrifying and scary in equal measure.

'We interrupt this programme to bring you an urgent news broadcast,' they say. 'Your world has changed and we thought you should know,' is what they mean.

What makes the 'We interrupt this programme . . .' announcement so thrilling is that it happens so rarely. They don't do it without a bloody good reason. They don't barge into *EastEnders* for any old news story. No, only the biggest and most impactful ones get the 'We interrupt . . .' treatment. Only the ones that make us stop, cry, think and reach for our loved ones.

Anyway, if you've never had it, then I'm afraid you've missed it. Apparently the BBC has stopped doing it. It's removed the 'We interrupt . . .' from its guidelines, and replaced it with something called 'an always-on approach to news broadcasting'. I wish it hadn't. I wish it'd introduced a 'usually-off approach' instead.

Since the Internet blew up we can't move for news. It's everywhere, it's inescapable and it's almost always bad. 'War!' it screams. 'Famine! Corruption! Rape! Climate change! Extremism! More war!' It's like being sprayed with an unending, unrelenting torrent of horse shit while being handcuffed to a radiator.

It's exhausting. But it's also – yep, you've guessed it – terrible for our mental health. Indeed, according to multiple studies, the more bad news we ingest the more depressed, anxious and angry we become. Certainly that's how it is for me. The more news media I ingest, the unhappier I am. Often just one article is enough to make me glum.

It reminds me of this Welsh pub that we used to visit as a family. It was a beautiful, serene spot with incredible views of Snowdonia. But what really made the place was the barman – an impossibly dour, perpetually grumpy man aptly named Dai (pronounced Die). To converse with Dai was to inject melancholy directly into your blood. It didn't matter how cheery you started a conversation, within two minutes Dai would have you reaching for the Prozac.

'Lovely weather,' you'd start out.

'Too bloody hot,' Dai would respond. 'I can't stand it when it's warm, see. Too many bloody bugs.'

Anyhow, that's how I feel about the press. It doesn't matter how chirpy I wake up, within a 30-second peruse of the news, I've got a frown like Frida Kahlo.

So what to do? Well, there are two options really. The first is that the media could just relax for a minute. They could go back to giving us the news at set times of the day. And turn down the volume when they do. Not everything is a 'crisis' or a 'national disgrace'. Not everything leads directly to Armageddon.

Sadly, something tells me that they're unlikely to go for this. Which leaves us with option two, namely that we can stop caring. Not totally, of course. After all, an active press is essential to democracy. But we could make little adjustments to minimise the amount of news-based turmoil in our lives. We could delete the apps, block the websites and switch over from Radio 4 to Magic FM ('more of the songs you love').

That's what I've been doing recently. Our flat has become a news-free zone. And boy has it cheered us up. Maybe, just maybe, no news really is good news.

It isn't all bad, by the way. Some of it's been bad, but mostly the Internet has been brilliant.

It's brought education to the masses. It's made knowledge free and available. It's helped topple dictators, prevent disasters and reunite loved ones. It's made the world smaller, but no less wondrous. It's brought us closer to nature, closer to understanding nature. It's introduced us to new cultures, places and people.

And it's made life easier. It's lifted the administrative burden of existence. We can order food when we want it, taxis when we need them, holidays when we can afford them. All at the click of a mouse or the tap of an opposable thumb. It's even tantalisingly close to eliminating the need for estate agents. Imagine that! Imagine a world free of estate agents. What a utopian nirvana that would be.

Of course the common retort is that, in making things easier, the Internet has made us lazier. And not just in terms of buying stuff. It's also, allegedly, made us lazy in other spheres. We can't be arsed to hang out together; we just text. We can't be bothered to meet each other; we just swipe. We can't be bothered to shag one another; we just watch porn. We can't be bothered to challenge ourselves; we just listen to opinions we agree with.

Sadly, all of these claims are substantiated with evidence. Digital communication *is* replacing face-to-face interactions. Dating apps *are* replacing bars as the place to meet a partner. We *are* watching a load more porn. And we *are* constructing ever-narrowing echo chambers for ourselves.

But somehow I'm not worried. Somehow, I'm still pro-Internet. Primarily because it is a *choice*. I feel like we've forgotten that. In our quest to blame everything on someone/something else, we've forgotten that lots of the Internet is optional. If we want to see our friends in person, or have sex with someone we love, or buy bog roll from an actual shop, or expose ourselves to a plurality of opinion, we can. No one's *making* us be crap. We're doing it to ourselves. And because it's elective, can't we just choose not to?

Some folks are. Growing numbers of people are giving up their phones, deactivating their social media accounts and embarking on a 'digital detox'. Which, according to the research, can be hugely beneficial. Even just four days without a phone has been shown to improve posture, sleep, mood and anxiety.

But surely a 'digital detox' is only a temporary fix. It's a week in The Priory followed by a crack and booze binge. What we need is something more sustainable, something more fundamental.

We need to stop texting, and start calling. We need to force ourselves out of the house, and out to the shops. We need to flirt properly, and love deeply. We need to visit places, see friends, and ask questions. We need to think. We need, put simply, a new normal. One where the Internet and technology complement the human experience, rather than replace it.

Getting there won't be easy, but it is essential. And it will be so worth it. Imagine being able to have all the benefits of the Internet, without any of the drawbacks. And imagine all of that, in a world without estate agents. Bliss.

WORKIN' 9 TO 5, WHAT A WAY TO MAKE YA MISERABLE

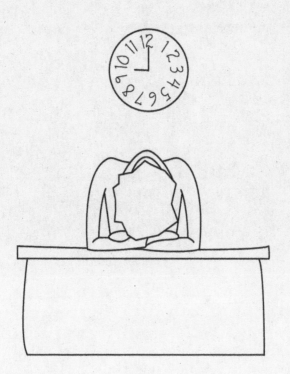

WORKIN' 9 TO 5, WHAT A WAY TO MAKE YA MISERABLE

MY FIRST JOB after university was as a management consultant.

Sounds fancy, I know. In some ways I suppose it was. It was reasonably well paid, and based in London, which was a plus. And it was for a big company that people had heard of. The sort of company that mothers boast about in Waitrose: 'I heard that your Rory got on to the accountancy grad scheme. You must be so terribly proud.' But it wasn't all roses. There were downsides, too. For example, I fucking hated it and was shit at doing it.

'Profitability and Cost Management' was the euphemistic name of my team. 'Sacking Nice People to Make Shareholders Rich' would have been more accurate. God it was wretched. And not just the bit where we sacked people. The mind-numbing quotidian nature of it also drove me to despair. The endless trains, planes, uncomfortable shoes, meetings, emails, PowerPoints, Premier Inns and DoubleTree by

Hiltons. It truly was a turd of a gig and I decided to leave after a year. I just couldn't take another day.

After a brief search, I decided that my next job would be selling advertising at a newspaper. It wasn't a decision informed by logic, so much as my desire to be a cool Don Draper character replete with Savile Row suits, hard liquor and loose morals.

Sadly, the reality wasn't quite what I'd imagined.

I doubt, for example, that Don Draper had Swedish techno music playing in his office. Or that he had to do 100 cold calls a day. Or that a good portion of those calls would culminate in him being told to 'fuck off'. And they really did tell me to 'fuck off'. Sometimes I deserved it (for example, the time I accidentally called someone while they were at their mother's funeral). But the strength of the animosity was nevertheless surprising. If you want to experience the deepest, darkest recesses of the human psyche, cold-call someone on a Monday morning and try to sell them advertising. I lasted two years flogging ads and then handed in my notice.

My next job was in a bank. Again, I've no idea why. It had something to do with marketing and I thought that sounded swish, and the money was good. But, man, was it boring. Oh my lord. It was interminable. So, so dull. It was like watching paint dry. No, worse – it was like watching cricket. I had nothing to do, and acres of time to do it. At one stage I got so bored that I started booking meeting rooms to watch Netflix. And then when my mobile data ran out, I took to sleeping in the toilets using a travel pillow made of loo rolls.

The weird thing was that I wasn't the only one behaving like this. Everyone was at it. Piss-taking took place on an epic scale. Colleagues would rock up at 11am and leave at 3pm. Or they'd take three hours for lunch on the basis of needing some 'time to think'. One colleague used to work from home 'without access to phone or email'. How does that work? That's not working from home, Steph, that's being on holiday.

I managed to eke out a year before handing in my notice, and taking a job back selling advertising. Why? I really haven't the foggiest. I guess I didn't have a better idea. If I'm honest, I still don't. I've spent a decade ricocheting from one job to the next, and am still totally clueless about what I should do with my life.

I wish I was cool with my lack of direction, but the truth is, I hate everything about it. I hate doing jobs that don't interest me. I hate doing jobs that I'm no good at. I hate not caring. I hate being bored. Above all, I hate not achieving what I thought I would.

On my current trajectory there's no way that I'll own a home or a car. There's no chance that I'll be able to give my (as yet unborn) children what I had. There's no hope that I'll be able to *provide*. Which sounds like an irrelevant, archaic throwback to the gendered bullshit of yesteryear, yet somehow isn't. I still see providing for my family as crucial to my success in life.

I've tried lots of things to get out of this career cul-de-sac, but escaping is harder than you think. For starters you can't change jobs too often without arousing employers' suspicion. So once you're in one, regardless of how unhappy it makes you, you have to stick it out for a bit.

Plus I need the money. Without a regular income I'd be broke quicker than you can say 'Job Centre Plus'. 'Couldn't you just dip into your savings while you job search?' you say. Pah! Savings?! Who do you think I am, a Saudi prince? A baby boomer? Between my Post Office savings account (thanks Mum) and my Help to Buy ISA, I've probably got enough dosh to last a month. And even that's pushing it.

There's social pressure, too. Ever since university I've felt the gaze of friends and family on my career. God knows how much unsolicited, shit career advice I've received over the years. 'You've just got to tough it out' they tell me with barely concealed schadenfreude. 'You don't want to quit within a year.'

Side hustles and projects have been a good distraction from the boredom. But, sadly, the relief has only ever been temporary. After a few weeks of planning they usually fall to the wayside. Like my idea to open a B&B in Crete. Or my scheme to sell falafel at festivals. Or my plan to sell ice cream from a boat by the beach. I got quite far with that one. The boat was to be called The Lolly Roger and we'd serve the best ices on the ocean. I even registered the company (Sir Francis Flake Holdings) and bought the web domain.

I know I'm not alone in all this; most of my friends have had, or are having, a job wobble. Even the ones who have trained for donkey's years – the architects, dentists and doctors – have started doubting their choices. Some have quit, some have retrained. Only one of my friends is still with the company he joined after university. And he's more miserable than me. After 10 years as an accountant he's got oodles of dosh, a flat and a car; and yet he still needs 100mg of Sertraline to get up every day.

I suppose some degree of career shuffling is to be expected now we're in our late twenties. The scramble to get a job after university was so fraught that most people took the first one they were offered. And now, 10 years later, folks are migrating towards gigs that they actually want.

But something more fundamental, more seismic, is also going on. It feels like my generation is much more professionally restless than those before us. We seem to be more demanding, more impatient. For our parents, a 'job' was a series of tasks that you did for money. That's not enough for us. We want those tasks to make us happy, too. And we want to do them on our own terms. We want to set our own targets, work flexibly and bring dogs to the office.

Some folks think it's because we're entitled, unwilling to graft and spoiled. I don't agree, particularly with the last one. My generation might have grown up with computers, but we're also poorer than our parents; more unemployed; more indebted; less likely to own a home; less likely to have a pension; more likely to be chronically lonely; and more likely to kill ourselves. How that qualifies as 'spoiled' is beyond me.

Instead, I think it's to do with our belief that there's always something better out there. We're plagued by this looming sense that the grass is always greener.

In my own case, I desperately hope that it is.

JUST A BIT OF
HARMLESS SELF—HARM

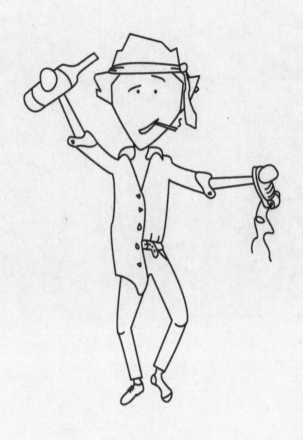

JUST A BIT OF
HARMLESS SELF—HARM

MY FIRST FEW years in London were brilliant fun. I loved getting to know the place, and revelled in my transition from out-of-towner to bona fide Londoner.

For all the misery at work, the money was welcome. Naturally I spent most of it on rent, and whatever was left went on new clothes and small lifestyle upgrades (branded tea bags, quilted loo roll, Pornhub Premium, etc.).

I was still living with friends, but it was different to when we lived together at university. London life had matured us, and accordingly our flat took on a pleasingly grown-up edge. We bought a swanky coffee table book, a proper cafetière and one of those room fragrance things with sticks. We even, in a moment of prodigal extravagance, hired a cleaning lady. Her name was Lina. We hired her purely because it rhymed with 'cleaner'.

ARE YOU A LONDONER?

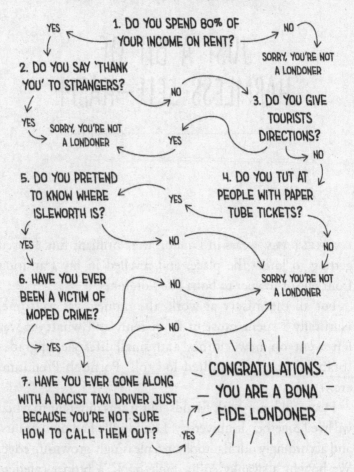

I partied hard. Partly because it was fun, but also as an escape from the ennui. Getting pissed was a fast track to creating memories, and a welcome (if fleeting) distraction from the boredom at work. So I did it loads. It started off as traditional binge drinking. I'd be sober all week, and then get mortally drunk on Friday and Saturday nights. But over time it grew to engulf the rest of the week, too.

Lots of the booze was paid for by work. One of the few reasons for joining the advertising industry is access to free, corporately-funded liquor. It's how they trick people into joining. 'Don't be a doctor or teacher,' they say, 'come and work in advertising. Your job will be pointless, but there will be a wine fridge in the office.'

But there was plenty of drinking at home, too. We always had beers in the fridge, and would think nothing of sinking three pints on a weeknight. Five if there was a pub quiz on. I can't tell you how many days started hungover. Definitely more than 50 per cent; probably it's closer to 80 per cent. I wasn't an alcoholic, mind you. I didn't need a drink, I just liked one. And compared to my friends and colleagues, my booze intake didn't seem that excessive. That was the problem.

Smoking was my other vice. I was good at cigarettes. I could roll them, light them in the wind and even blow perfect smoke rings. I used to light up whatever. It didn't matter if it was raining or if I had a chest infection. If there was a ciggie to be smoked, I'd be smoking it. I was getting through a packet a day by the time I quit.

Exercise in my early- to mid-twenties was strictly prohibited. I can't remember doing it at all. Perhaps there was the odd game of squash, or the occasional, furtive free trial at the local Fitness First. But I certainly wasn't working out regularly. Why would I bother? I was far too busy getting pissed, smoking ciggies and being hungover to go running.

It was around my twenty-sixth birthday that things began to unravel. It started with a prolonged period of poor sleep. Then, over about six months, I started to get very down in the dumps. There were even a couple of panic attacks. I found them terrifying, but not enough to slow down. Instead I tried to explain them away. I'd been burning the candle at both ends, I told myself. Things would get better. It was nothing that I couldn't handle.

Occasionally I'd take it easy for a few weeks, lay off the booze, commute from ciggies to vaping. But before long, the boozing, smoking and unknowing self-harm would resume.

Taking all this together, it seems so obvious that trouble was brewing. The warning signs were there. I just happened to ignore them.

I wish dearly that I hadn't. I wish that I'd listened to my body.

I wish that I'd heard my mind's screams for help. I wish I'd cut down on the drinking. I wish I'd stopped smoking. I wish I'd quit the jobs I hated sooner. I wish I'd abandoned social media. I wish I'd recognised how toxic masculinity was affecting me. I wish I'd realised how my family history predisposed me to mental ill health. I wish, more than anything, that I hadn't tipped myself over the edge.

But I didn't. I thought I was invincible.

I wasn't.

RECOVERY'S A ROLLERCOASTER

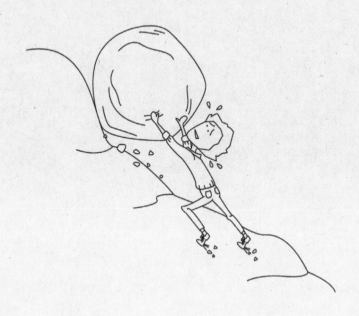

RECOVERY'S A ROLLERCOASTER

AS YOU MAY have spotted, the title of this bit is a play on Ronan Keating's hit song 'Life is a Rollercoaster'. There are two reasons for this.

The first is that the music of Ronan Keating occupies a place in my heart labelled 'things I love because my mother loves them'. Other residents of this cardiac nook include *Downton Abbey*, gardening and the cooking of Yotam Ottolenghi. At least I think it's Yotam Ottolenghi who my mother likes – it's hard to be certain given that her pronunciation changes every time she says it: 'I've done an Ottolengthy salad', 'It's Ottoslunging flatbreads for dinner', 'Do you like the pears? They're an Ottovonbismark.'

Anyway, I wanted to include Ronan somewhere to make my mother smile, and this felt as good a point as any.

The second, more obvious, reason is that recovery *really is* like a rollercoaster. It's up and down, left and right, fast and then slow. Except, unlike a rollercoaster, recovery doesn't end. It's not a finite experience, or a set period of time. It's a process – a messy, unpredictable and non-linear one. Some days I'm good, others I'm awful. The one thing I never am is cured.

People always ask me that. 'Are you cured?' 'Are you fixed?' No, I'm not. I'm much, much better, but my anxiety is still there. The episodes are shorter and less intense, and the distances between them have grown. But they do still happen. Involuntary, obsessive anxious thoughts still whirr around my head. From time to time I can't sleep. I still practise certain compulsions. I still get really, terrifyingly down.

What's different, however, is that I now know it's only temporary. In the past I didn't. I thought that every bout of anxiety, every tsunami of depression, would last forever. I thought that it would never get better. But it did. It does. *It always gets better.*

The first year after my breakdown wasn't about recovery, it was about survival. It was 12 months spent enduring the anxiety, and learning to live nervously. I worried, I worried about worry, and I developed the compulsions. There were a few good days in that first year – Cali and I had a couple of great holidays – but mostly they were bad.

My attitude at the time oscillated from complete capitulation to the thoughts, to a desperate desire to get better. One minute I'd be crying hopelessly in the toilets at work. The next I'd be googling radical treatment options, searching frantically for a cure.

I had no way of knowing which state of mind I'd wake up with. And, beyond developing my list of bizarre rituals and compulsions, I wasn't taking any real, positive action. It was an awful year. I worried constantly, slept little and cried loads.

I also talked about my anxiety a lot. I was forever crowbarring my thoughts into conversations with friends. It was a validation and reassurance thing. I wanted them to tell me that I was normal, and that I'd get better soon. 'My friend Paul had exactly that,' I longed for them to say. 'It took a few months but he's totally fixed now.'

Plus it was the only thing that I had to talk about. Having an anxiety disorder was the only thing I had going on. I hadn't been up to much, I didn't know how work was going, I hadn't watched the football. All I had was my anxiety. I was a one-way street, a conversation cul-de-sac, a handbrake on chit-chat.

Things got better when I changed jobs.

This was the move from the boring bank, back to selling advertising. I hadn't expected it to make much of a difference, but it did. It was exciting to meet new colleagues, learn new tasks and raid new stationery cupboards. And, for about a year, that excitement proved sufficient to banish my anxiety. Not totally, of course. Most days it was still switched 'on'. It's just that, for the first time since my breakdown, there were occasional days when it was turned 'off'.

Irritatingly, whether I'd awaken with it turned 'on' or 'off' was anyone's guess. And the transitions from 'off' to 'on' – the relapses – were both unpredictable and brutal. It didn't seem to matter where I was, or what I was doing, my brain would simply decide to 'go anxious', and that was that.

It happened at weddings, dinner parties and even, once, during a performance by Cirque du Soleil. There I was, cheerfully gawping at the sexy French-Canadian acrobats, when – BANG! – the worries returned: 'You're going to forget to breathe', 'You're going to spend your life worrying about breathing', 'Why are you so fucking useless?'

There was also no predicting how long a relapse would last. Sometimes I'd snap out of it after a few hours. Usually it was a few weeks, maybe a month. A month 'on', a few days 'off', another two weeks 'on', a day 'off', three weeks 'on' – that's how it was for the second year.

Then things changed. Firstly I started getting stuck into CBT. And secondly, my attitude shifted. I made the conscious decision to stop obsessing over a cure, and accepted that my recovery would take time and be non-linear. I started seeing relapses as necessary hurdles to jump over, rather than as evidence that I was a shit person. Above all, I came to believe that my anxiety would pass.

Throughout Year One I'd thought that my anxiety would never get better. Year Two showed me that it would. And Year Three was about applying that discovery. 'You've been this bad before and got better,' I'd tell myself. 'So don't worry, this won't last forever.'

Probably the best analogy for my recovery is the process of taking a flight. Year One was the take-off – it was loud, bumpy and (if you hate flying like me) very scary. Year Two was the cruise, albeit a very turbulent one. I did have some fleeting moments of smooth flight, but mostly the seatbelt signs were illuminated and the cabin crew were definitely not serving coffee. Year Three (which brings us up to the present) has been the landing. I haven't touched down properly yet, and there have been plenty of bumps on the way down, but I'm nearly there. I can see the ground. I can envision stepping off the plane. I can imagine a life without anxiety.

I still despise my condition. And I still get terrifically down about it. Even though my anxious episodes are shorter, more spread out and less intense, their arrival still makes me sad. The feeling of being 'normal' is such bliss, and it hurts to lose it. Of course I'm grateful to have had it at all. I just wish it could have stayed. It's like going back to school after the holidays – I'd be thankful for the summer, but sad that it was over.

Naturally, the longer I've been free of anxiety, the worse the sadness is. Relapsing after a long period of being 'cured', is always more painful than a short one. It's the last whack around the head; a final, humiliating kick in the groin from a bullying condition that says 'How dare you think that you're cured?' It's pernicious like that.

The big difference between the past and the present is that I have a plan.

In consort with the CBT therapist, I've developed a list of things that usually make it better. And I've also got much more adept at detecting when an anxious episode is inbound.

The trick is to identify which worrisome thoughts are legitimate (don't forget – some things are worth worrying about), and which thoughts are illogical inventions of my anxiety disorder. For example, worrying about taking an exam is probably legitimate. Whereas worrying about forgetting to breathe is not.

The problem is that my anxious, illogical thoughts present themselves as legitimate concerns. Ergo, I don't know which thoughts are worth worrying about and which require action. Or at least that's how it used to be. These days I'm much better at spotting anxious thoughts. I've learned how they work. I've studied their disguises and deceptions. I can recognise them from a distance, pick them out of a crowd. It's like spotting an old friend from the gait of their walk, the tone of their laugh or the scent of their fabric softener.

For example, thoughts that are involuntary, repetitive and incessant are usually anxious ones. Genuine worries and concerns don't present like this. They're more fluid, they come and go. In contrast, anxious thoughts just go round, and round, and round, and round.

Worries about worry are the second 'tell'. 'Normal' people don't worry about worry. They worry, sure. But they never go that extra step. For instance, while most people would have a worrisome thought like, 'I might miss the train', only people with an anxiety disorder would think 'I'm never going to enjoy life because I'll always be worrying about missing the train.' The transition from first- to second-order worry can be extremely subtle. But if I am able to notice it, I know to activate my anti-anxiety plan.

Another handy tool is the 'are you completely fucking mental?' test. It's fairly simple: I imagine saying my thoughts out loud, and envisage what my friends would say. If their response would be 'fair play', then that's a sign that a worry is legitimate. If it's 'are you completely fucking mental?', then it probably isn't.

One of the only good things about anxious thoughts is that they follow patterns. They're creatures of habit. This is a good thing because it helps me to identify them. I know, for example, that my condition is always worse in the morning. For whatever reason, my mind is at its most eccentric during those first few waking hours. Knowing this enables me to be on high alert for anxious thoughts in the morning. If it's an incessant worry and it's in the morning, it's usually driven by my condition rather than something genuine.

Finally, anxious thoughts do a weird thing when I'm out and about. I'm not sure how to describe it – it's a kind of projection. I'll be walking down the street and I'll try to project my worries onto the strangers around me. So when I wasn't sleeping I'd look at random passers-by and question whether they'd slept the night before. And if so, how well? What did they do differently to me? Do they think about sleeping as much as I do? Do they worry about it? And so on. Very peculiar, but also very useful. Because whenever I catch myself doing this, I know for sure that I'm either in an anxious episode, or heading for one.

Having spotted that anxiety is inbound, the big question is what to do about it. The next few sections are all about this, and I don't want to spoil your appetite, but, generally speaking, it's about being kind to myself. I tone down any drinking or partying; I dial up exercising; and I engage my CBT techniques.

I also go into my phone and find the note where I record my worries. For three years I've jotted down my anxious thoughts in my phone. It's my journal of misery, my diary of desperation. All my worries are there, catalogued neatly, like an episode list for some dismal series on Netflix. There are the ones about not sleeping, and not breathing, and dying alone, and getting a sore throat, and being nervous for my whole life.

The note is titled 'Don't Worry, be Hapy' [sic].

I wish it wasn't. 'Don't Worry, be Hapy' is such a crap title. It's misspelled and lazily uncorrected, not very funny and not quite ironic. In my defence, I never thought that it would see the light of day. And, besides, I don't go to 'Don't Worry . . .' for its witty title; I read it to be reminded of the many, many, many times when I've been bad and then recovered. Even better are those records showing when I didn't think I would recover, but did. They're incontrovertible, weapons-grade evidence with which to fight the thoughts in my head. And because it's written down even my ninja-level anxious brain can't argue with it.

Which is half the battle. Actually, it's the whole battle. If I can remind myself that *it always gets better*, even when I think that it won't, I'm nearly there. As Rudyard Kipling nearly wrote, 'If you can remember that, then you'll be a non-Anxious Man, my son!'

HELP! I NEED SOMEBODY

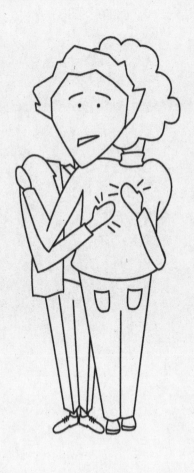

HELP! I NEED SOMEBODY

THERE WERE LOTS of reasons why I didn't want to tell my parents about my breakdown.

I felt shame and embarrassment about being weak, obviously. And I was afraid that they'd panic, or think that they'd done something wrong. They hadn't. In fact, throughout my life, they'd done everything *right*. They'd given me a brilliant, warm childhood. They'd encouraged me through school and exams. They'd been there during work woes, break-ups and house moves. They'd been fantastic parents and I couldn't bear the idea of them feeling guilty. So I kept quiet and tried to put a brave face on things.

I lasted for two weeks. I couldn't conceal it any longer than that. I couldn't go it alone another day. I needed my parents' and my family's help, love and support. I needed *them*.

Of course when I did tell them, they were phenomenal. My parents understood the problem immediately, and my brothers, cousins and friends all huddled around me. They helped me to get help, they occupied my weekends, they came to London and took me out for dinner. My brother and cousin even let me sleep in their office.

Odd, I know. But when my insomnia was really bad it became the only place I could sleep. There was something so comforting about their passive company. Just having them there was enough to help me drift off. So after a sleepless night I'd lie to my boss that I was working from home, walk over to their office, find the sofa in the corner and nap. Usually it was only an hour or so. That was all I needed. An hour, asleep, surrounded by love.

I'm sure my brother and cousin thought I was utterly bonkers, but if they did, they didn't show it. They made it seem like the most normal thing in the world. And it made me feel so much better. Not just the sleep, but the affirmation and reassurance from them. Then again, that's the simplicity of unconditional love. It isn't showy or loud; it's quiet and understated. It isn't always visible, but it is always there. It supports you when you're down and smiles with you when you're up. It's the best insurance policy that money can't buy.

Strangers, too, have been brilliant with me. Like the lady in A&E who bought me a Mars bar because she thought I looked 'gloomy'. Or the taxi driver who saw me crying and gave me the fare for free. Or the nurse who gave me some sleeping pills even though she shouldn't have.

At one stage it seemed I couldn't move for spontaneous acts of human kindness. It even happened after a spinning class. I remember it vividly because it was the first time I'd tried spinning, which, in case you don't know, is a trendy exercise fad built around indoor cycling. There's loud music, flashing lights and an instructor who shouts meaningless motivational nonsense like 'Pump your energy!', 'Be your vibe!' and 'Make tomorrow today!'. Anyway, we were just coming to the end of the class when I started chatting to the bloke next to me.

'How come you started spinning?' he asked.

'I had a mental breakdown about a year ago and am hoping that it will help,' I overshared.

'Shit, sorry to hear that,' said the stranger. 'I had a similar thing last year. Let's grab a beer after this.'

Quite amazing, seeing as I'd only known the guy for five minutes. We're quite good pals now. His name is Matt.

I suppose my point is that people are amazing. All you have to do is ask for help, and most folks will. They'll give you just the right help, in just the right quantities and at just the right times. All without agenda or prejudice. They'll do it simply because they care.

It's not easy, mind you. People with mental health problems can be bloody hard work. Stewing in our thoughts all day can make us negative and self-centred, as well as boring and changeable. One second we want X, the next we're demanding Y. Having a mental health problem can also change people, and that's difficult for friends and family. Extroverts can become introverts; senses of humour can disappear overnight.

It's tough. But that's what humans are for. 'Tough' is where we do our best work.

The hardest part of supporting someone with anxiety or depression is knowing what to say. 'I want to say the right things and make it better, but I'm scared of saying the wrong things and making it worse.' I hear this all the time.

In light of this, I've put together this little guide. It's by no means complete, but hopefully it's a good starting point. But, first, two caveats:

1. As you'll see, I've done it through the hackneyed use of 'Dos and Don'ts'. I appreciate that this is quite *Good Housekeeping* ('Our dos and don'ts for the perfect napkin swan'). I just couldn't think of another way. Sorry.

2. I'm very conscious of being overprescriptive – these pointers are just what's worked for me, and if you want to go rogue then please be my guest.

Do

1. Ask the question
As you know, my first job after university was firing people for money (aka management consulting).

As part of the 'onboarding' process for this miserable role I was sent off to a hotel in the Cotswolds, along with about 500 others, for two weeks of intensive training. It was a sort of 'Business Bullshit 101' – somewhere between an episode of *The Apprentice* and a terrorist training camp. We were taught everything from how to do PowerPoint presentations, through to Japanese business etiquette and how to run a conference call.

Naturally, given that the thing was run by management consultants, every module was dripping in meaningless corporate buzzwords. People didn't do things; they 'actioned' them. We couldn't think; we had to 'dive deep'. They weren't presentations; they were 'deliverables'. Then there were the endless feedback sessions. Jesus. You couldn't do a poo without first conducting a quick peer-to-peer feedback session ('I'd like to see you flush faster next time, Simon'). Except, of course, they weren't called 'feedback sessions' because that opened up the possibility of negative feedback. So instead they were called 'great because . . . even better if . . .' sessions.

It was excruciating and pointless. And yet, for all my railing against it, there are some bits of the training – vapid little platitudes usually – that I still remember today. One of which is that phrase 'If you don't ask the question, the answer is always no.'

I like this phrase a lot. It works perfectly for mental health. If you don't ask your friend or colleague or child how they are, then you'll never know. And if they mumble something incoherent, or say they're fine when you know they're not, don't worry. Don't push. Don't pry. You've asked the question. They know you're there. They'll talk to you if they need to.

2. Believe them

We live in exciting times for mental health. People are starting to talk about it, the media is starting to cover it and
politicians are even talking about maybe doing something
about it. All of this is terribly good news, but there's also a
downside. Namely, that increasing numbers of people are
becoming increasingly sceptical. 'Oh she's got depression?
How very convenient.' Or 'Anxiety? Pah! We all get nervous
sometimes!' That sort of thing.

There are two reasons why scepticism is unfounded.

Firstly, for all the signs of positive change, life is still easier
without a mental health problem. Folks with depression,
anxiety and OCD are still discriminated against. I can't see
why people would opt in for that. And secondly, even if a small
number of people *are* pretending, isn't believing the liars a
price worth paying for believing the true sufferers? I think it is.

There's nothing worse than not being believed. It
happened to me loads at the start. Lots of people thought I
was making it up. They thought it was a phase, or that I was
being a hypochondriac. I wasn't. It was real. It was awful. It
also sounded bizarre and unlikely (particularly to my friends
who had never had a mental illness), but I promise that it
was real.

If someone tells you that they're struggling, believe them.
It's the first step to becoming helpful.

3. Do your thing

This is a very simple piece of advice, but it's also one of the
most important: not everyone can be everything. Different

friends give me different things. Some of them I go to for sympathy, some I call for advice and some I see for good, old-fashioned fun.

So before trying to help someone it's worth considering your strengths and weaknesses. What do you bring to the party? Are you naturally sympathetic, or would it feel forced? Do you have personal experience to inform your advice, or would it largely be guesswork? Does the person need a kick up the arse, and are you the person to deliver a cold hard truth? And so on.

You alone will know where you can help out most, and you mustn't feel down if that role isn't Chief Sympathiser. Chief Advice-Giver and Chief Arse-Kicker are just as important. The main thing is that you identify your role and do it.

4. Be nice

If the last bit of advice seemed simple, then I'm positive that this bit will have people shouting 'Well obviously, you donut!', but I'm going to say it anyway. My number one piece of advice for supporting someone with a mental health problem is: be nice. Which is a limp, flaccid and meaningless phrase – it's linguistic mild Cheddar, literary Coldplay. And yet, it's also the perfect descriptor for what I'm after.

Be nice. Not amazing, not brilliant, not fantastic. Just 'nice'. Just do the basics of friendship, but really, really well. Call them. Text them. Listen. Care. Remember. Be thoughtful. Invite them to things. Introduce them to people. Above all: be patient. Because, sometimes, people with mental health problems can make lousy, tiresome mates. We can be late, tired, forgetful, irascible, snappy, self-absorbed. We can forget things. We can forget *you*. We can want to talk about it one minute and then not want to talk about it the next. We can be laughing at a party but then crying in the Uber home. We can, quite simply, be an arse ache.

But importantly, we're only an arse ache for a while. We get better, *it gets better*. So be patient. Over time, slowly, unsteadily, your old friend will re-emerge. And it will have been so worth it.

Don't

1. Get it wrong

I say the wrong things all the time. Not 'wrong' in the moral sense, just in the 'well now I look like a plonker' sense. Like the time I finished a client call with 'Love you, bye', or the time I called my boss Dad.

I'm also terrible at remembering names. Case in point: I spent all of 2017 calling my colleague Kat, Sophie. Even now it makes me cringe. I only found out when they gave me my leaving card.

'Who's Kat?' I asked the guy next to me.

'You know Kat!' he said. 'Blonde hair, wheelchair.'

'Bugger.'

Then there are the occasions when I've said the right thing, but to the wrong person.

'I think Emily Stanley wants to get with me,' I tried to text a friend.

'No I don't,' Emily replied.

My point is: it's painful and embarrassing to say the wrong things, but that's about it. Nobody dies when you say the wrong thing. Nobody calls the cops. Yes, there's a danger of getting it wrong, but there's also a huge upside if you get it right. Certainly the rewards outweigh the risks.

That said, there are a few common mistakes worth considering.

For example, the best way to avoid saying the wrong things is to say relatively few things. You don't need to take a monastic vow of silence, simply do more listening than talking. They want you to listen. So do that.

Also, never say anything with the word 'cheer' in it. That means no 'cheer up', no 'reasons to stay cheerful', no Cheerios. Because when someone is in a pit of despair – be it an anxious, obsessive or depressive one – the very last thing they want to be told is to 'cheer up'. If they could cheer up, they would. They can't. That's why they're talking to you. So you can leave your 'cheer' at the door – you're not in *Bring It On* now (Go Toros!).

Reassurance is a tricky one. In the short term it can seem like the right thing to do, but in the longer term it can make it much worse. The problem is that there are 'diminishing marginal returns' to reassurance. The more you do it, the less meaningful it becomes. So if you can, I'd suggest avoiding it entirely. Or if you really do want to reassure someone, make it general rather than specific. The answer to 'Will I get better soon?' should be 'Most people get better', rather than 'I'm sure you will get better tomorrow.'

THE REASSURANCE TRAP

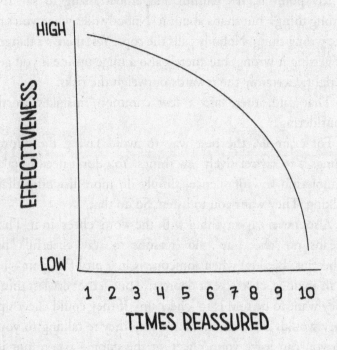

The same is true of facilitating or enabling compulsions. Allowing or helping someone to perform their rituals might make life easier initially, but over time it has the opposite effect. Because by facilitating the compulsion you validate the obsession, and the OCD knot gets tighter.

That's how it was with my sleep-related compulsions. At its worst there were tons of things that I had to do before bedtime – shower, read, drink certain amounts of water, control breathing, go to the loo, lie in a certain position, etc. If I couldn't do one of these things I'd go to pieces.

Seeing how much distress it caused me, Cali used to go out of her way to help me. If we were booking a hotel, for example, she'd make sure that the bed was big enough, or that there was a shower. And when I went through a phase of sleeping on the floor, or when I refused to sleep in the same room at all, she'd say that she didn't mind, that lots of couples didn't share a bed.

Of course, it all came from a place of love and kindness and support. She wanted to help me, to prevent me from feeling panicked or scared. The problem was that in helping me to do all the little things, she reinforced the logic in my head. It made me think that my entirely illogical worries were legitimate. And as the weeks went on, it got worse and worse.

Eventually she had enough. The list of pre-sleep chores got too long.

'I think this is becoming a bit much,' she said. 'Do you think we could try not doing it for a few nights and see what happens?'

So we did. For the first week it was very uncomfortable, and I didn't sleep a whole lot. Then one evening I slept like a dream, and that was it. I had proven, with Cali's help, that the rituals were just obsessive inventions. I didn't need to do them any more. I was free. I haven't slept on the floor since.

In challenging me, Cali set me on the road to gaining control over my mind. If you find yourself in a similar position, I'd consider doing the same. It's delicate work, obviously. So tread carefully and, like Cali, consider nesting the challenge in a question. For some reason, question marks make everything feel less pushy.

The only other recommendation is to not say anything belittling. 'We all get nervous' is a common annoyance. As is 'Oh you've got a mental health problem, how trendy.' You wouldn't say that to someone with cancer or heart disease (the next biggest killers of men under 45). So do me a favour and don't say it to us either.

2. Give up

Helping someone with a mental health problem isn't hard work. It can sound like it is, but it isn't. I know this from speaking with others, and because I've done it myself. The truth is that being there for someone at their lowest ebb, helping them through a crisis, seeing them on the road to recovery, feels great.

Of course there will be moments of frustration. There will be times when someone seems to be getting better, only to then get worse. Or when they don't listen, or won't talk. But hang in there. Because the feeling you get when you make a difference is just incredible. That's the only cool thing about mental health problems: you don't need lots of specialist training or equipment to be useful. You just need to be alive. You just need to be *there*.

Do
- Ask the question
- Believe them
- Do your thing
- Be nice

Don't
- Talk more than you listen
- Say anything related to 'cheer'
- Blindly reassure or facilitate
- Trivialise
- Give up

EAT, PRAY, LOVE . . . AN EARLY NIGHT

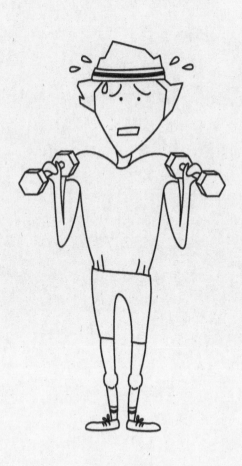

EAT, PRAY, LOVE . . . AN EARLY NIGHT

I'VE HAD A weird relationship with booze ever since my breakdown.

Throughout all this, my biggest fear has been returning to those first few weeks after *that fucking party*. Just thinking about the constant panic, the mental turmoil and insomnia makes me shiver. And given that my problems started after an evening on the sauce, it seemed sensible to give up drinking as a precaution. So I did. For a year I became completely teetotal.

Why only a year? Two reasons. Firstly, wedding season kicked off in earnest and I just couldn't face another reading of 1 Corinthians 13 without a drink. And secondly because I came to realise that stopping drinking entirely wasn't healthy.

That might seem odd, especially given how settled the science is regarding liquor and mental health, but it's true.

Because before my mental wobbles I was quite capable of having a hangover without also having a breakdown. I spent a good chunk of my twenties being hungover and I managed to bumble along just fine. Therefore, my decision to stop drinking wasn't driven by a physiological necessity; but rather by a psychological fear. And when you look at it in those terms, stopping drinking was just another compulsion in response to another obsession. It was the same as having to go to the loo twice before turning out the light, or the need to drink exactly five litres of water a day. It sounds counterintuitive, but I was doing a good thing for a bad reason. Changing the bed sheets is an ostensibly good thing, but not if you're covering up for having eaten a curry in bed (I have definitely not done this).

It took me about a year to fully relax the rules around drinking. The first few furtive lagers after sobriety were the scariest. It's pathetic, I know, but I fully expected that first Heineken to send me spiralling, back to square one. It didn't, of course. And neither did the second, or third. Slowly my relationship with drinking began to normalise.

Having said that, I do still try not to get terrifically pissed. But that's less because of psychological fear, and more because my sobriety taught me how fantastic unhungover weekends are. If I haven't been hammered drunk I can get up at 8am on Sunday and do stuff. I can go to the gym, or play squash, or read the newspaper. I can do hobbies, see friends and have fun. The weekend becomes my oyster. I can go anywhere, do anything. Just last weekend I was up so early that I was actually the first person in the IKEA car park. Imagine that. Imagine being able to have 12 Swedish meatballs with lingonberry jam, alone, at 10am on a Sunday. Life just doesn't get better than that.

The tricky thing about drinking less is having to talk to drunk people. Sorry, I know how sanctimonious and awful that sounds, but it's true. Drunk people are annoying. They just are. They talk gibberish, and shout, and bump into you. Or they fall asleep, or start fights, or initiate 'deep and meaningfuls'. That's probably my worst type of drunk person. Actually, no. By some way, the argumentative pseudo-intellectual drunks are the worst – that bloke who says 'just playing devil's advocate . . .' before introducing some shit argument, supported by invented facts. I played witness to this at a dinner party a few weeks ago.

'Just playing devil's advocate,' said the drunk man called Rupert, 'isn't there an argument that says, like, look, Jimmy Savile did some terrible things, but, like, shouldn't we let sleeping dogs lie?'

No, Rupert, there isn't. And no we shouldn't.

The other hard thing is not being smug. This is easier than it sounds, although I might have transgressed earlier re: IKEA at 10am. Mostly, however, I'm pretty good at it. I never say, 'Wow you were really drunk last night' or 'How many wines did you have?' or 'I expect you're hungover.' I try not to get annoyed when Cali wakes me up, humming of Prosecco. And I never talk about how good I feel. No one wants to know how pious I've been, or how much weight I've lost, or how much extra money I seem to have. So I try to keep my trap shut.

Curiously, I'm not the only one taking it easy with booze. Loads of people seem to be cooling off. Young people, especially, are hanging up their drinking boots. Indeed, since 2005 the number of 16- to 24-year-olds living as teetotallers has increased by 60 per cent, while the percentage of them drinking to excess has halved.

There are lots of theories about why this is happening. It could be because booze is too expensive for the cash-strapped Gen Zs. Or it could be that attitudes towards booze have changed and people are more health-conscious than ever. There's even research in America which suggests that it's all about social media. Where in the past teenagers rebelled by getting pissed, now, the research suggests, they do so by posting seditious content online.

Either way, the societal slide towards sobriety has got to be a good thing. Particularly for mental health. Not only does drinking make us sleep less and worse, it also plays havoc with our brain chemistry. And not in the ways you might think. Lots of people think of booze as *either* a depressant *or* a stimulant. But, in reality, it's both. Alcohol slows certain neurotransmitters like glutamate and GABA, but at the same time boosts levels of dopamine. The combined effect of these opposing forces is that, as Katy Perry once sang, 'You're up then you're down, you're in then you're out.' Put simply, alcohol creates imbalance and that makes us feel depressed and anxious.

The other positive of everyone drinking less is that it's becoming more socially acceptable. Five years ago, I would have been laughed out of the pub for ordering a lemonade.

It isn't like that now. People are much more open to it, primarily because they're trying to cut down themselves. Even in my old industry – advertising – folks are taking it easy. Naturally there are still a few old soaks drinking claret at lunch and eating roast swan, but they're becoming increasingly rare. Job interviews never take place in the pub any more and client entertainment is much more abstemious.

Perhaps it would have been harder to quit partying if I'd been any good at it. That's what made it difficult when I stopped smoking – it felt perverse to walk away from something that I was so good at. With partying it was the opposite. I've never really liked clubbing, or raving, or anything exciting like that, so putting a lid on it hasn't been very hard. I do like a pub though. But that's OK. I can still go to the pub; I just tend to leave a little earlier. I have two pints rather than five. I still get to laugh, smile and enjoy my friends. I just also get to enjoy an empty IKEA car park (note to self: must stop going on about IKEA).

Despite having the body fat precentage of prosciutto, I've always had a go at sports.

I'm usually pretty crap, and I don't tend to last very long, but I do love the excitement of competitive sport. As well as the opportunity to buy all the gear. For evidence of this, you need only look in the cupboard under our stairs where, among the suitcases and cleaning materials, you'll find tennis racquets, hockey sticks, shuttlecocks, football boots, rugby balls, gum shields and even the odd golf club.

All of them barely used, some of them still in the packaging.

Sadly, though, having the equipment does not a sportsman make. I never score goals, or make important tackles, or throw things far enough. I've only scored a try once. And I've lost count of how many times the wind blew me over in my hockey goal-keeping pads. God, that used to be mortifying. There I'd be, flailing around on the AstroTurf, like an upturned crab, while the opposition dribbled the ball past me and scored. 'Fuck's sake Roberts!' said the captain. 'Stay on your fucking feet.'

I've done much more sport since my breakdown. Sport and the gym. Probably three times a week I'll lace up the old Asics and go for a run, or lift some tiny weights. And I can't tell you what a difference it's made. Not to my body, of course. I'm still a lard-arse. I still walk that thrilling line between 'normal' and 'overweight' on the BMI chart. And, although there has been a fractional increase in the size of my right arm, that's less to do with the gym and more to do with the solitude of writing a book.

Exercise does all manner of good things for our mental health. Most notably, and in contrast to boozing, it's brilliant news for brain chemistry. People who exercise tend to exhibit higher levels of the 'happy chemical' serotonin, for example. And they get to enjoy more endorphins – the lovely neurotransmitters responsible for that delicious post-exercise surge. Taken together, these chemicals seem to make us much cheerier. Either they do it directly or they improve our mood, which, in turn, makes us happier. Regardless, the more of these chemicals we get, the better.

HOW DOES EXERCISE AFFECT BRAIN CHEMISTRY?

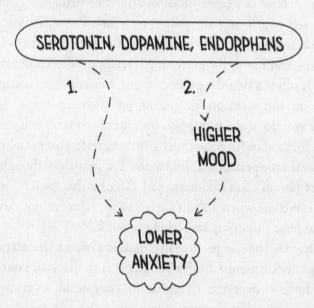

SEROTONIN, DOPAMINE, ENDORPHINS

1.

2.

HIGHER MOOD

LOWER ANXIETY

Exercise is also really good for sleep – it helps us fall asleep quicker, sleep longer and enjoy better quality slumber. One of the reasons is all about changing body temperatures. Humans sleep better when we're a bit colder (a hangover from our outdoor, cavepeople past), and as we approach bedtime our bodies reduce in temperature by about one or two degrees. Cooling down after exercise mimics this effect and as a result we sleep better. Pretty neat.

Exercise also helps to establish our circadian rhythms, and has been shown to reduce arousal. Not that sort of arousal, you dirty bugger – the anxious or depressed sort. All of which is ruddy good for snoozing.

But physiology aside, the most important thing that I get from exercise is a sense of self-worth. I've struggled greatly with self-worth over the past three years. I've spent lots of time hating myself – for being weak, for worrying, for being down – and I find that exercising is really good at countering this. It offers a singular point of focus, something to concentrate on and a reason for getting up in the morning. The more you do it, the better you become. Each time you run a little further, or lift something a little heavier, you get a little boost. It's the perfect antidote to the 'I'm so useless' thoughts: 'I just ran an extra kilometre so I can't be that useless' or 'I just exercised when I didn't have to' or 'I'm feeling down but at least I'm doing something about it.'

That last one is particularly handy. One of the scariest things about mental health problems is the lack of control you have – over the thoughts in your head, over what happens next, over whether you get better or worse. It's terrifying. Through exercise, though, I can regain some control. It's a lever to pull, an item to add to the 'positives' column: 'OK, I have this problem but I'm taking action.'

I've experienced all of these benefits. I feel at my best, my most vital, after running or lifting some weights. I also feel chuffed every time I do it, and rewarded every time I get a smidge better. And my sleep has got much better, too.

It wasn't easy at first. Finding the initial motivation was tough. But also, for the couch potato, gyms are daunting places; all those grunting muscle men and lithe marathon mums can be very intimidating. That's why I only used the running machine in the first year. I'd sneak my way into the gym, creep over to a treadmill, do my little run and potter home. But after a few months that got deathly dull, and so I decided to take on the weights bit. Not on my own, obviously. I raided my Help to Buy ISA once more and enlisted a snooty personal trainer to show me the ropes. Or rather, the weights.

I'm still no good at the gym. I still haven't got anything approaching abs or pecs. I still wheeze, heave and splutter. I still sweat. I mean *really* sweat. Not a thin, sexy film of perspiration; full-on, Darth-Vader-in-a-sauna sweat.

In a way, though, that's missing the point. I don't exercise because I'm good at it; I do it because I *need* it. And because I enjoy it. Not always, naturally – about once a month I have a stinker of a session and wish I'd never gone. But mostly I feel like I'm in a Nike advert – it's just me, my goals and my 'Go Girl' playlist.

What's cool is that you don't need to exercise loads to feel the benefits. Three times a week, for a period of 10 weeks, seems to be the going rate. And while rhythmic aerobic exercises appear the most effective (e.g. running, cycling, swimming), even light exertion can also have an impact. According to one study just walking briskly for 10 to 15 minutes a day can have a positive effect.

IT'S THE REMIX TO COGNITION

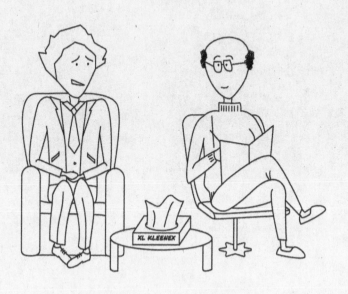

IT'S THE REMIX TO COGNITION

IT'S 9:10 ON a Tuesday morning and the man sat opposite me has his eyebrows furrowed.

'I'm sorry, Josh, but I'm not sure I follow,' he says quietly in a soft Northern accent. 'I don't see the connection between eating pasta and dying alone.'

'Because pasta brings on the anxiety, which means that I won't sleep, which means that Cali won't sleep. And she's not going to want to go out with someone if they stop her sleeping. So she'll dump me and I'll die alone,' I say with frustration. 'What connection can you *not* see?'

'Well,' he responds calmly, 'it's a convincing chain of events, but have you ever eaten pasta and not become nervous?'

'Yes.'

'And have you ever been nervous but still slept?'

'Yes.'

'Or have you ever not slept, but Cali hasn't dumped you?'

'Yes.'

'OK, so do you think that there's a chance that you could eat pasta and not die alone?'

'Well, when you put it like that . . .'

So went the typical CBT session at the start of my recovery. The chap sitting opposite me, Brian, is the second of two CBT therapists I've seen. He's a slim man, maybe a tad shorter than me, with a broad grin and glasses. He's also calm, unassuming and Northern. I think his accent is Middlesbrough, but that's only a guess. I don't know for certain. In fact, I don't know anything about Brian for certain. That's not why we're there, he tells me. Our meetings aren't about him or his life. And whenever I try to move the conversation towards him, he gently massages it back to me.

I suppose it's a sensible policy, but it does make for an odd asymmetry of information. Brian knows everything about me – from the last time I watched porn (three months ago), to the last time I cried (three months minus two seconds ago) – while I know nothing about him: I don't know where he lives, if he's married or if he has kids. Last Christmas I bought him a bottle of wine without realising that he's teetotal.

Oddly, though, I don't mind. I trust Brian implicitly. I guess there are contractual obligations to ensure confidentiality, but even without them I'd still tell him everything. He's that sort of bloke. His whole demeanour screams 'You can tell me anything and I'll take it to my grave.' I'm the opposite. My demeanour screams 'Tell me anything and it will be on Twitter before sundown.'

I also don't mind because it works. Telling Brian everything makes me feel better. After I say it, we pick it apart and usually by the end of our hour-long session I feel much, much happier.

At its heart, CBT is a simple set of techniques for challenging the thoughts in our heads.

It starts from the premise that our thoughts, emotions and physical feelings are all interconnected. Thoughts lead to emotions, which lead to physical sensations, and vice versa. Just as anxious thoughts in our heads can raise our heart rates, so too can a raised heart rate lead to anxious thoughts.

The aim of CBT is to interrupt this process by isolating and challenging the logic of the thoughts. If you can prove the thoughts to be invented rubbish, then you can prevent the emotional or physical responses from taking place. You still have the thoughts, you just don't care about them. You go from playing in the rugby game, to watching from the sidelines.

At the start, it was a manual process. I used to spend hours clunkily isolating and challenging the thoughts in my head. It's a bit like presiding over a mental courtroom. Every time a worrisome thought popped into my head, I'd try to catch it and cross-examine it. Where was the evidence that I'd forget to breathe again? Wasn't there loads of evidence to the contrary?

Initially I would have to go into a different room to conduct my 'thought trials'. But, over time, the mechanics of CBT have become automatic. Nowadays, I can do it in the background. Brian's list of 'thinking errors' is a big help. Thinking errors are mental mistakes that our brains make. I've summarised my most frequent ones below. (I've used my anxiety around sleeping to highlight how they work as I imagine that is the most universal.)

Naturally, not all my thought trials lead to successful convictions. From time to time my brain concocts a worry so convincing that I can't pick it apart alone. That's when I need Brian's help. He's a far better prosecutor of thoughts than me. He's the Judge Judy of shitty thoughts.

We also discuss more theoretical stuff – the role of anxiety in human evolution, the ways that anxiety can be useful, brain chemistry, and so on. The idea being that, as Marie Curie said, 'Nothing in life is to be feared, it is only to be understood.'

One model that I particularly like is the somewhat unimaginatively titled 'Anxiety Equation'. It's a simple way of establishing why different thoughts inspire different levels of anxiety. By understanding *why* we fear some things more than others, we're able to start challenging that fear. In the equation there are two factors that increase anxiety – perceived likelihood of a worry coming true, and perceived 'awfulness' if it does – and one factor that reduces anxiety – our perceived ability to cope.

THE ANXIETY EQUATION

$$\text{ANXIETY} = \frac{\text{LIKELIHOOD} \times \text{AWFULNESS}}{\text{LIKELIHOOD TO COPE}}$$

The scariest thoughts are those which are very likely to happen, very bad if they do and for which there is no capacity to cope. I'm struggling to think of a good example of these. Maybe the thoughts you get when your plane crashes?

I use the anxiety equation as a way of reducing the potency of my thoughts. There are three ways that I do this: I question the likelihood of a thought coming true; or I explore how awful it would really be; or I look into my ability to cope. Often one of the factors is fixed, but that's OK. If that's the case, I just focus on the other two.

For example, dying alone as a result of insomnia would be pretty awful. But in the face of this fixed 'awfulness' we can focus on the other two factors: likelihood and ability to cope. Is it really likely that I'd get dumped for not being able to sleep? Isn't there loads of evidence to the contrary? And at the same time, isn't there a ton of evidence to suggest that, even if I did get dumped, I would be fine? Haven't I been dumped many times before, and survived?

Common thinking errors
Black-and-white thinking
WHAT IT IS: Thinking in terms of all or nothing.

EXAMPLE: 'I didn't sleep at all last night.'

HOW TO CHALLENGE:

- Did you really not sleep at all?
- Didn't you sleep a bit, maybe for a few minutes or hours?

Mental filtering

WHAT IT IS: Only paying attention to certain types of evidence.

EXAMPLE: 'I didn't sleep last night, so I will never sleep again.'

HOW TO CHALLENGE:

- Isn't there lots of evidence that you will sleep again?
- What's the worst that can happen if you don't?

Overgeneralising

WHAT IT IS: Drawing broad conclusions from narrow evidence.

EXAMPLE: 'I didn't sleep last night, so everything is awful.'

HOW TO CHALLENGE:

- What else exactly is awful?
- And how awful is it really?

Catastrophising

WHAT IT IS: Reaching horrific conclusions based on little evidence.

EXAMPLE: 'If I don't sleep tonight Cali will dump me (because she won't want to share a bed with an insomniac), so I will die alone.'

HOW TO CHALLENGE:

- How many times have you not slept and not been dumped?
- Why will tonight be so different?
- What would Cali say if you said this out loud?

Labelling

WHAT IT IS: Assigning unhelpful labels to yourself/people.

EXAMPLE: 'I didn't sleep last night therefore I'm a useless piece of shit.'

HOW TO CHALLENGE:

- Why?
- Aren't you simply a person who didn't sleep?

Blaming

WHAT IT IS: Assigning personal guilt.

EXAMPLE: 'It's my fault that I didn't sleep last night.'

HOW TO CHALLENGE:

• Why? Millions of people suffer from insomnia.

Should/must

WHAT IT IS: Assigning expectations (realistic or otherwise) to create invented standards.

EXAMPLE: 'I should have slept better last night. I must sleep to be considered normal.'

HOW TO CHALLENGE:

• What is 'normal'? And who decides what is 'normal'?

• Why does being 'normal' matter?

Another very helpful thing that I did with Brian was create an anxiety map. He told me to imagine a scale of nervousness from 0 to 10, and to record whenever I felt more than a 5. I was to write down what I was thinking about, what emotions were attached to it and any physical sensations that I was experiencing. Being an insufferable tosser, I went straight to Paperchase and bought a small, leather-bound notebook. I was going to carry it in my breast pocket like some romantic, melancholic poet jotting down my worries with ink and quill. That lasted for two days before I lost the £10 notebook down the back of a train seat. That's when I created 'Don't Worry, be Hapy'. I imagine that, were they alive today, Byron and Shelley would have done the same.

As well as providing me with an invaluable point of reference when I'm having a wobble, the mapping exercise was also extremely instructive. It revealed that, although there was a great deal of randomness to my anxiety, there were also some undeniable patterns.

It was always worse towards the start of the week, for example. Or after more than a couple of evenings of drinking (even if it was very low-level boozing). Or after three days without exercising. It was also negatively correlated with my fulfilment at work – the less I had to do from 9 to 5, the more anxious I was. Conversely, if I had a project on it was always better. It didn't particularly matter what the project was – studying for an exam, sorting out the garden – but having an 'extracurricular' seemed to make a difference.

By recording all of this I was able to start taking action based on fact, rather than conjecture. Before I was obsessively doing this or giving up that based on a single piece of evidence (i.e. whatever happened last time). Now I was able to look at the patterns over many months and base my actions on multiple pieces of evidence.

Writing everything down also uncovered how bizarre my thoughts were. Often just seeing them in writing was enough to make me realise how illogical they were. It helped me to put some distance between me and the thoughts. If you've never done CBT you probably still think that your involuntary thoughts are 'you'. They're not. They're just involuntary thoughts. They come from somewhere in your brain, but they're not a reflection of your personality or what you truly think or believe. Writing them down and analysing them helped me to realise this.

Seeing Brian, and doing CBT, made a speedy and profound impact on my anxiety. I found this surprising.

Before I came to depend on it, I thought that CBT sounded like a load of mumbo jumbo – the sort of psycho-babble claptrap you'd expect from a wacky aunt in a tie-dye kaftan. And not just because the idea of 'talking yourself better' seemed so hopelessly boho; I also thought that the setup of therapy felt hideously self-indulgent. What could be more egomaniacal than paying someone to listen to you talk about yourself?

I had all manner of preconceptions about what went on during therapy. I envisaged thick carpets, modern art and a black leather chaise longue. Brian's office isn't really like that. It's a shabby little place in a higgledy-piggledy building in London's financial district. The best thing about Brian's office is the tiny church and courtyard that sits behind it. As churches go, this one is very low-fi, but it's still a lovely spot to sit and collect my thoughts after each session. The peace-ful courtyard, covered as it is in pigeon poo, serves as a welcome halfway house between the cosy confines of ther-apy and the brutal realities of life.

Almost immediately after meeting Brian I started to feel better, or better equipped at least. CBT has provided a useful and effective framework for working at my condition. I'm not alone in this. The evidence base for its efficacy, particu-larly for anxiety disorders, is large and growing. Some experts even call it 'the gold standard'. I agree wholeheartedly, although there are a few things worth considering – a few top tips – to get the most from CBT.

The first is that you don't necessarily need a therapist. You can absolutely learn the techniques from books, or websites, or podcasts. Obviously, you have to be sure that you're getting the good shit, but I see no reason why you couldn't work through a programme at your own pace, in your own home. Most of CBT is homework anyway – writing things down, conducting thought trials – so it would just be more of that.

However, if you do choose to go down the therapist route, it's imperative to shop around. Most people don't. I didn't. Before Brian I spent a year seeing this other bloke even though we never clicked and he repeatedly forgot my name.

The right therapist is someone who you can trust, obviously. But also someone who you feel comfortable being challenged by. You have to be interested in their opinions. You have to want to listen to them. Which doesn't mean that you need to like them, or have much in common with them. On the contrary, I think one of the reasons that Brian and I work so well is because we have almost nothing in common. As a result, my conversations with Brian have introduced me to new opinions, broadened my world view and even led to me questioning some of my basic truths.

I remember one conversation about money in particular. I had been approached for a new job, which seemed interesting, but would have involved taking a fairly hefty pay cut. This, in turn, was driving a whole load of anxious thoughts (e.g. 'If you take this job you will die alone because no one wants to date a loser who takes a pay cut').

'It's interesting that you place so much importance on money,' Brian said. 'Why do you think that might be?'

The answer was obvious. From the moment I arrived at boarding school I'd been drilled in the importance of money. Jobs don't exist to make you happy; they're there to make you rich. We needed to earn more than our colleagues, more than our friends, more than our parents. Careers, like life, were a competition. Only losers pretend otherwise.

Brian didn't see it like this. Gently he suggested that life needn't be a competition, and that, even if it were, money wasn't a very good way of keeping score.

'You have a well-paid job,' he said. 'Would you consider yourself to be winning?'

In about five minutes we undid 20 years of social conditioning. And that wouldn't have been possible if Brian had the same background as me.

'Yah mate, completely agree,' he would have said. 'Money is, like, yah, pretty bloody great.'

It's also important to realise that the right therapist for one person might not be right for someone else. Everyone's conditions, circumstances, personalities and outlooks are different. Different people need different things. There are simply far too many, highly personalised variables.

A similar thing is true of cost. All too often people equate cost with quality. They think that the pricier the therapist, the better their therapy. It doesn't work like that. Spending loads of cash won't guarantee that a person will click with another person. Therapists found on the NHS can be just as good as the super-duper, million-pounds-a-minute ones on Harley Street. I found Brian through Google. Just find someone who works for you.

Therapist or no therapist, for CBT to work you have to commit to it. You have to be open-minded and you have to do what you're told. If you have to keep a diary, then do. If you have to read something, then read it. Actively use the techniques, even when they feel silly or when you can't see how they will help. Have faith that they will. Because they do. I'm evidence of that. And I'm not the only one.

CBT also takes time. I felt some impact immediately, but it wasn't until a few months had passed that I really noticed the difference. And when it did start to work, the anxious thoughts didn't disappear; I just noticed myself caring less about them. To reiterate, CBT isn't about stopping thoughts popping into your head, it's about not losing your shit when they do. It's about having a thought like 'I could die alone' and that being the end of it. That's how it's been for me. I still get the thoughts, I just don't always believe them, and I don't get any of the other stuff either – the dry mouth, tight chest, raised heart rate and knotted stomach.

Achieving this took time, which isn't surprising. It took me 26 years to get into this mess, so it'll take a good few more to get out of it.

A final, important note of caution is that CBT can occasionally be uncomfortable. In order to confront and challenge anxieties, I have to think about them. Which is easy if I'm going through a bad patch – the thoughts will be at the front of my mind, and I'll be desperate for help. But if I'm in a good patch, if I'm free of worry or depression or obsession, I don't want to think about my unhappy thoughts. I don't want to jinx it. I don't want to talk about them, for fear of bringing them back. I want to let sleeping dogs lie. I want to carry on as though none of this ever happened.

I've cancelled two sessions as a result of this logic. Both times I've regretted it. Both times I've felt disappointed at myself for caving in in the face of a worry. The whole purpose of doing CBT is to free myself of nervous and compulsive behaviour. Cancelling therapy sessions is the opposite of that. It's giving in; it's allowing the thoughts in my head to dictate the way that I live my life.

Of course, as my condition has improved, I've tapered the amount that I see Brian. It used to be weekly, now it's every three months or so. But I have sworn never to cancel a session because I'm 'going through a good patch'. After all, if I'm having such a brilliant time, why would I be worried about seeing a therapist?

THE DRUGS DON'T WORK
(AT LEAST NOT FOR ME)

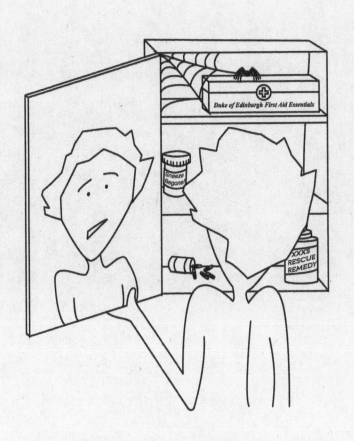

THE DRUGS DON'T WORK
(AT LEAST NOT FOR ME)

PILLS AND I do not go well together.

I've never taken the recreational ones, and I'm slightly terrified of the prescription ones. Mostly I'm scared of dependency. I hate the idea of *needing* something, of relying on a pill to get me out of bed. I'm also fearful that, if I did take pills to manage my anxiety, they'd blunt my existence, or render it pointless. Like all great movies, life is best enjoyed in glorious technicolour, on a huge screen and with the sound turned up. And I worry that anti-anxiety medication would reduce my experience to the grainy low resolution feel of a pirated DVD, or a dodgy download. Of course, I might be wrong.

It is because of these fears that I've never taken antidepressants. I've been offered them loads, sometimes quite insistently. One doctor in particular wouldn't take no for an answer. The whole experience reminded me of afternoon tea with an overzealous granny.

'Do have another egg sandwich Josh.'

'I'm fine thanks.'

'Go on Josh, *have another egg sandwich.*'

At first I was surprised to be offered antidepressants. Naïve as I am, I thought that they were only used to treat depression. In reality, they're prescribed for all sorts of conditions, and they can be terrifically effective. I know lots of people who swear by them. I've just been too fearful of the potential side effects to give them a try. I've got plenty of worries to be getting on with already, I certainly don't need to throw a potential drug dependency into the mix.

That said, I haven't been completely drug-free, particularly when it comes to insomnia. Frankly, after three consecutive sleepless nights I'd do almost anything in return for some sleep. I'd happily lick the floor, or eat a kangaroo's bum hole. Whatever you want, I'll do it. And that includes the short and infrequent use of sleeping pills.

I've tried two types: Valium and Zopiclone.

Valium sleep isn't really sleep; it's the land of the living dead, the 'sleeping awake'. For three weeks I took 5mg of it before hopping into bed (after fluffing the pillows, before doing the breathing, at the same time as sipping the water). It tastes bitter and soapy, a bit like raw cranberries (if you've ever been stupid enough to eat some).

The first sign that the Valium is kicking in, for me at least, is a slight swaying sensation. I'm lying perfectly still, but it feels like I'm being slowly rocked from side to side. Then my heartbeat becomes slower and deeper. It's not quieter, just lower in pitch, almost like my blood has thickened and become harder to pump. I know I'm getting close when I feel sweat on my forehead. From there it's usually only a few minutes before I start dipping into and out of sleep. Which is how it stays for the remainder of the night. A night on Valium is a night spent on the fuzzy edge between wakefulness and sleep. And when I do sleep, it's invariably interrupted by that weird sensation of falling. Valium sleep is hot, fevered and bitty.

Zopiclone is a different ball game. If Valium is the living dead, then Zopiclone is the 'dead dead'. It's complete anaesthesia. And it's quicker. It tastes like licking a copper coin, but within minutes I'm gone. I don't dream. I don't wake up in the night. I don't remember anything in the morning. For eight hours I'm effectively deceased. One of the things that worries people about death is not knowing what happens next. Where do we go? Heaven? Hell? I reckon we go to the same place after dying that I go to when I take Zopiclone: total nothingness; complete, oblivious unconsciousness.

As well as the odd sleeping pill, I've also occasionally taken beta blockers.

They're very clever pills, beta blockers. As the name suggests, they block the stress hormones (adrenaline, noradrenaline, etc.), and in so doing make us feel less nervous. As in, you actually *feel* less nervous. The heart rate is lower, the stomach is unknotted and breathing remains normal. I still think the worrisome thoughts, my body simply doesn't respond. It's quite bizarre. I've had moments when my head is in complete turmoil and yet, with my

40mg of Propranolol on board, my body behaves like it's lying on a beach.

Perhaps because of their effectiveness, there's a rather grim industry growing up around beta blockers. Online pharmacies – some of them very trendy – are in the middle of a big sales push. Not only for clinical anxiety disorders, but also as a 'cure' for any of life's little nervous moments. 'Worried about your big date?' reads one digital advert. 'Propranolol can help stop your shaky voice, sweating and racing heart-beat.' All of which is technically true, but also a bit creepy.

Because where does it end? If we start taking pills for first dates, what will we medicate for next? Meeting the parents? Getting married? Parenthood? Life is to be lived, not 'managed' or 'cured'. And, besides, human emotions are delicate things. The sensations of 'nervousness' are almost identical to 'excitement'. No pill – no matter how clever – can eliminate the former, without also dulling the latter. And who wants to live an unexciting life? Isn't that the whole reason we're here? Isn't that the whole fucking point?

Of course, I'm not suggesting that folks flush their pills down the loo. Absolutely not. If they work, and if the doctor says crack on, then you'd be mad not to take them. It's just that, from my own experience, and from speaking to others, it seems that pills are unlikely to be enough. Most recoveries will involve other stuff. For me that's been drinking less, exercising more and practising CBT. But I've also spoken to people who swear by yoga, or moving to the countryside, or swimming in cold water. My favourite one, however, came from my former boss's boss, Helen.

Helen is a formidable lady, with an imposing demeanour and a reputation for not suffering fools (she once described a colleague as 'a waste of oxygen'). She's also had GAD since her twenties. Helen's condition is so quintessential, so archetypal, that I imagine it's written down in a textbook somewhere. It's GAD sent straight from central casting. It's the Ronseal of mental health problems – it does exactly what it says on the tin. Namely, Helen worries about everything. She even, just like me, worries about worrying.

What's different about Helen isn't her illness, it's her recovery. She tried all the usual stuff, of course, but the thing that really made a difference was getting a dog.

The idea of getting a pet to cheer oneself up is neither new, nor novel. In fact, the concept of pet ownership dates back to Palaeolithic times. It started off as a working relationship, a partnership, between dogs and humans – the dogs helped the humans hunt, and in return the humans fed the dogs and kept them warm. Then, as the millennia wore on, we became rather fond of our canine colleagues and started domesticating them from birth. Thus pet ownership was born.

Nowadays it's called Animal-Assisted Therapy (AAT), and Helen is convinced that it's improved her anxiety. And she's not alone. According to one recent survey, a whopping 75 per cent of pet owners reported mental health improvement as a result of their pets.

I love the idea of AAT. Mostly because I'm desperate to get a dog, but also because it's a therapy based on warmth and affection, rather than brain chemicals and cognitive restructuring.

It's so simple and beautiful: you love the pet, the pet loves you, everyone gets happier. What could be better than that?

As theories go, the serotonin one is pretty neat. 'Anxiety and depression are caused by a lack of serotonin in the brain,' it says. 'Increase serotonin, and you cure the anxiety and depression.'

It's an elegant, easy-to-grasp explanation, and one which is hugely popular with the public. Indeed, over 80 per cent of people believe that chemical imbalances cause depression. And it's little wonder that pharmaceutical companies have made untold riches on the back of this premise.

The only problem with it is that, well, it's total rubbish.

At best, the serotonin theory is overly simplistic. Most probably, it's complete bullshit. That's what the research tells us, as well as the man who first proposed it – a chap called George Ashcroft. He's on record as saying that *the link between serotonin and mental health, doesn't exist.*

So why does the theory continue to enjoy such prominence?

Certainly, a big part of the theory's success is its simplicity. Simple explanations always capture the public imagination better than complicated ones. Just like a car needs its oil topping up occasionally, some people's brains need a little extra serotonin. Can't argue with that.

Then there's the fact that a good chunk of pharmaceutical company profits rests on the theory being correct. Or being believed to be correct. Selective Serotonin Reuptake Inhibitors (SSRIs) are the most widely prescribed antidepressants on earth. And their use depends on the serotonin insufficiency idea being true. So the pharma companies have spent ungodly quantities of wonga ensuring that everyone believes it. Not only us punters, but doctors and governments too. If you think I'm lying, google 'Prozac marketing' and prepare to be amazed.

Which isn't to say that SSRIs don't work; they do. Some of them work very well. They just don't work by topping up serotonin. Which is, I guess, the only thing that matters. If SSRIs make a difference, if they make people happier, then that's all that matters.

Except it does feel like we're missing a trick by not demanding more from the people who make our pills. At the moment we're settling for medication that is grounded in a debunked myth, and which works through some mystery mechanism. And I think we deserve better than that. But we're not going to get it until we stop believing this 'serotonin imbalance' twaddle. We need to move beyond that. We need a proper scientific framework for mental health. And we need to accept that it's likely to be very complicated. Because brains are complicated. That's why they're so brilliant.

LOVE IS THE DRUG

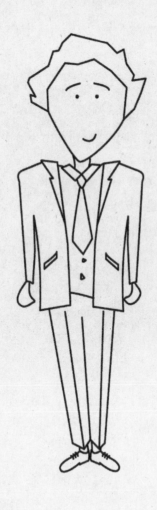

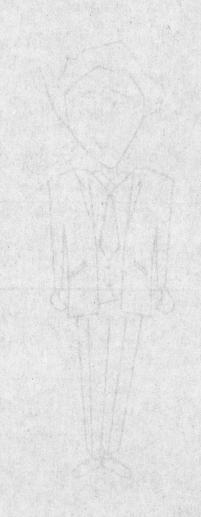

LOVE IS THE DRUG

I'VE ALWAYS RATHER enjoyed dating: the expectation, the nervous excitement, the potential for a sexy outcome, and the validation. Particularly given my porky childhood, it's affirming to have someone accept the invitation to date.

'She has agreed to *Gone Girl* at the Ritzy,' I can tell myself. 'I can't be *that* unsightly.'

And, anyway, who doesn't enjoy a good, hard flirt?

The dates in my mid-twenties were the best. Teenage dates were thrilling, seat-of-the pants stuff. And the ones during university were blissfully pseudo-bohemian ('Come round for *The Notebook* and a spliff?'). But the mid-twenties ones were somehow better. Maybe it was because the girls expected more; sharing a cigarette or buying them a late-night shawarma was no longer enough. They wanted extra, and I enjoyed rising to the occasion.

There was Annie the teacher, Maddison the lawyer, Celia the doctor. There was even a French student, Amélie, who couldn't speak any English. Without a shared tongue we

183

relied purely on body language, pheromones and animalistic instincts to communicate. Which might sound sexy, but was actually pretty awkward. Stilted reruns of my GCSE French oral exam don't make for a great date (*Pour mon anniversaire j'ai reçu un vélo rouge*). There were other duds, too. The girl who'd recently been released from prison ('She was asking for it'), for example. Or the girl who was writing an unauthorised biography of Ken Livingstone (pro tip: do not bring up Israel on a first date). Or the girl who said she was a lesbian just after I'd taken my shirt off.

'But we've been talking about your ex-boyfriends all evening and snogging,' I said.

'Yep,' she said, scanning my wobbly torso, 'definitely a lesbian.'

In total, I've told four girls that I loved them. Only one of them was a lie. Awful, I know. If I told you that it was on the first day of a week-long staycation, perhaps you'd forgive me.

'I love you,' she said as we departed London.

'Oh fuck,' I thought. 'I love you, too,' I said.

I shouldn't have. I was racked with guilt for weeks. And it made the subsequent break-up much harder: 'But you said you loved me?'

I resolved never to lie about being in love again. Thankfully, I won't have to. Barring some serious cock-up, I think I've fallen in love for the last time.

I met Cali at a dinner party in Fulham. It was a setup by our friends Harry and Gemma. We'd both been single for a while, and I think they took pity. So a sham birthday dinner was improvised, a shoddy paella was cooked (sorry Harry) and some Jacob's Creek was unscrewed.

Cali was wearing a stripy T-shirt and denim dungarees. A sort of 'kids' television presenter chic'. She had long, blonde hair which fell naturally to one side, brown eyes and a very broad grin. Which, as it happens, is her signature move. Of the 960 minutes in any normal waking day, Cali spends circa 959 of them smiling. I was taken with her immediately and, over the course of that evening, my life changed.

It's difficult to describe the sensation I felt that evening. Half of it was pure elation, utter joy at having found someone so brilliant. But there was also a terrifying reality that she might not feel the same; that my infatuation could go unrequited. For the first few months it did. Cali proved a terrifically, beguilingly tough nut to crack. I tried all sorts – we went to galleries, to dinner, to the cinema, and still she wouldn't snog me. I even went to sodding Glastonbury in a bid to woo her. Although that was my fault really. I should never have said that I liked festivals.

'Which ones are you going to this summer?' she asked.

'Err . . .' I said while grasping around my brain for the name of *any* music festival.

'Glyndebourne, no, wait, err, Glastonbury?'

'Amazing!' she said. 'Me too!'

The moment I got home I set about finding a ticket, which, as you might know, is near impossible. The festival was only three weeks away, and tickets had been sold out for nearly nine months. By some miracle, however, I did find

ANXIOUS MAN

someone who'd sell me one as long as I rented his caravan. I said yes immediately. It was the most expensive thing I've ever bought (and I've bought vegetables from Whole Foods), but it was also my only option. Either I coughed up the cash or kissed goodbye to Cali. I undertook yet another raid of my Help to Buy ISA and texted Mum: 'Please could you post my wellies to London?'

Is there anything better than the start of a relationship? The flirting, the laughter, the showing off to each other. That magical stage of exploration when you're learning each other's lives, hopes and habits. When you're meeting each other's friends and families, gently absorbing their world into your own. Gradually you build your lives together. The glasses of wine, the sharing pudding, the laughing in bed, the walks to the train station. You share showers, and cook dinner, and talk incessantly. You think about them incessantly. You text them incessantly, each time agonising over exactly what to say. Love washes over both of you. They come to depend on you, and you on them. Before long they are you, or a part of you at least. After a few weeks, maybe months, you say 'it'. You've felt it for a while, but needed to be sure. Now you are. You tell them. They say it back.

If it hadn't been for Cali – for love – I might have killed myself at the end of Year One. That might sound melodramatic, but it's true. I was just so down, so worried, so desperately unhappy. But then she saved me. Lovely, smiley, funny, clever Cali with her unique blend of tough and, well, normal love. A generous helping of 'You need to

186

pull yourself together because you're scaring me' with a good blob of 'Come on, let's go to the gym.' She pushed me to get better, and gradually I did.

Love is the foundation on which I've built my recovery. Without it, the main pillars – exercise, lifestyle changes, CBT – would have crumbled long ago. I suspect it's the same for everyone who's had a breakdown, or has a mental health problem. Discover love if you can – be it romantic, platonic or familial – and you discover the solid key to recovery.

People often ask me, particularly since I was given the opportunity to write this book, whether I'm glad that it happened to me. 'Now you get to live your dream of writing a book,' someone said to me recently. I could see their logic, but my answer was – and remains – a big, fat, completely unqualified 'no'.

In no way am I grateful for my breakdown. It's been the worst thing ever to happen to me. It's given me sleepless nights, Zombie Days and so much more besides. There have been some good days and, recently, there have been many more good days than bad ones. But taking it all together I'd still give anything for a time machine.

The only positive, aside from this book, is that I've become a better person. 'Better' is such a bland, ordinary, banal word. But that's exactly the sort of change that has taken place. I haven't become a radically better person. I'm not reformed, reinvented or reinvigorated. I'm the same mildly overweight, middle-class man that I was before. I'm just a tad more caring, a smidge more empathetic. I send my friends congratulations cards when they get engaged, and flowers when they're ill. I volunteer at Mind. I help the lady next door with her shopping. Last week I even lent someone my drill, no questions asked – 'Bring it back when you can' – which is a pretty big deal. It's a fancy Bosch one with lots of attachments and its own little briefcase.

When I studied Economics we were taught to consider all human beings as 'rational actors'. People, we were told, make decisions by weighing up all the different options and choosing the one which is most valuable to them. This was a lie. There are lots of reasons why humans make decisions, but almost none of them are rational.

None more so than the decision of my friends, family and colleagues to help me. What do they stand to gain? What's in it for them? How do they benefit from my happiness? Where's their reward for talking to me, or sitting with me in the cinema, or letting me sleep in their office? The only person who is behaving remotely rationally is Brian. And even his decision runs counter to his own self-interest – with his compassion, wisdom and patience he could be making a fortune in the corporate world. Instead he chooses to help people.

No, human beings are inherently *irrational*. But that's what makes us so brilliant, so beautiful. Before my breakdown I took this for granted. I was down on humans. These days it's hard *not* to be down on humans. Being a horrible, self-centred, haterist is de rigueur. Being a tosser is 'in'. And during times like these it's easy to write each other off, to flip the bird and turn away. My breakdown, and the way people have treated me, is a constant reminder not to do this.

People are incredible. You just have to let them be incredible. You have to give them permission. Write them a chit – 'Please help me' – and most of them will. They'll support you, love you and help you get better. And you *will* get better. It will get better.

Because it always gets better.

NOTES

Why Me?

Mind, 2016. Understanding mental health problems. Retrieved from https://www.mind.org.uk/media/3244655/understanding-mental-health-problems-2016.pdf.

Sheline, Y.I., 2011. Depression and the hippocampus: cause or effect? *Biological Psychiatry*, *70*(4), p. 308.

The Shame Game

Breen, J. and Shoko, T., 2007. Suicide is a social not an individual problem: Japan in International Perspective. *The Asia-Pacific Journal | Japan Focus Volume*, *5*(8).

Chambers, A., 3 Aug. 2010. Japan: ending the culture of the 'honourable' suicide. The *Guardian*. Retrieved from https://www.theguardian.com/commentisfree/2010/aug/03/japan-honourable-suicide-rate.

Wingfield-Hayes, R., 3 Jul. 2015. Why does Japan have such a high suicide rate? *BBC News*. Retrieved from https://www.bbc.co.uk/news/world-33362387.

World Health Organization, 2018. Suicide rates (per 100 000 population). Retrieved from https://www.who.int/gho/mental_health/suicide_rates/en/.

Man Up, Break Down

Hewitt, R., 30 Apr. 2018. Mental health discovery. Retrieved from https://digital.nhs.uk/blog/transformation-blog/2018/mental-health-discovery.

McVean, A., 31 Jul, 2017. The history of hysteria. *McGill University*. Retrieved from https://www.mcgill.ca/oss/article/history-quackery/history-hysteria.

Office for National Statistics, 18 Dec. 2017. Suicides in the UK: 2016 registrations. Retrieved from https://www.ons.gov.uk/peoplepopulation-andcommunity/birthsdeathsandmarriages/deaths/bulletins/suicidesin-theunitedkingdom/2016registrations.

Science Museum. Brought to life: Mental health and illness. Retrieved from http://broughttolife.sciencemuseum.org.uk/broughttolife/themes/menalhealthandillness.

Worldwide Worry

American Psychological Association, 1 Nov. 2017. Stress in America: The state of our nation. Retrieved from https://www.apa.org/images/state-nation_tcm7-225609.pdf.

Taylor, C., 13 Feb. 2019. Online dating isn't a game. It's literally changing humanity. *MashableUK*. Retrieved from https://mashable.com/article/online-dating-change-world/?europe=true.

Time Magazine, 2012. Your wireless life: Results of TIME's mobility poll. Retrieved from http://content.time.com/time/interactive/0,31813,2122187,00.html.

Watson, E., 14 Oct. 2014. Pornography addiction among men is on the rise. *Huffington Post*. Retrieved from https://www.huffpost.com/entry/pornography-addiction-amo_b_5963460.

Workin' 9 to 5, What a Way to Make Ya Miserable

Hobbes, M. Why millennials are facing the scariest financial future of any generation since the Great Depression. *Huffington Post*. Retrieved from https://highline.huffingtonpost.com/articles/en/poor-millennials/.

Nova, A., 25 Oct. 2018. Waiting longer to buy a house could hurt millennials in retirement. *NECN*. Retrieved from https://www.necn.com/news/business/Waiting-Longer-to-Buy-a-House-Could-Hurt-Millennials-in-Retirement--498567691.html.

Roberts, Y., 29 Apr. 2018. Millennials are struggling. Is it the fault of the baby boomers? The *Guardian*. Retrieved from https://www.theguardian.com/society/2018/apr/29/millennials-struggling-is-it-fault-of-baby-boomers-intergenerational-fairness.

Watson, P., 25 Sep. 2018. Real wage growth is actually falling. *Forbes*. Retrieved from https://www.forbes.com/sites/patrickwwatson/2018/09/25/real-wage-growth-is-actually-falling/#5ab411b67284.

Eat, Pray, Love . . . An Early Night

Ekkekakis, P., Hall, E. E., VanLanduyt, L. M. and Petruzzello, S. J., 2000. Walking in (affective) circles: can short walks enhance affect? *Journal of Behavioral Medicine*, 23(3), pp. 245–75.

Horne, J. A. and Staff, L. H. E., 1983. Exercise and sleep: body-heating effects. *Sleep*, 6(1), pp. 36–46.

Human Animal Bond Research Institute, 2016. Survey: Pet owners and the human–animal bond. Retrieved from https://habri.org/2016-pet-owners-survey.

Lin, T. W. and Kuo, Y. M., 2013. Exercise benefits brain function: the monoamine connection. *Brain Sciences*, 3(1), pp. 39–53.

Mental Health Foundation, 2006. Cheers? Understanding the relationship between alcohol and mental health. Retrieved from https://www.mentalhealth.org.uk/publications/cheers-understanding-relationship-between-alcohol-and-mental-health.

Mental Health Foundation, 2018. How to . . . Look after your mental health using exercise. Retrieved from https://www.mentalhealth.org.uk/publications/how-to-using-exercise.

NHS, 10 Oct. 2018. Young people turning their backs on alcohol. Retrieved from https://www.nhs.uk/news/lifestyle-and-exercise/young-people-turning-their-backs-alcohol/.

Passos, G. S., Poyares, D., Santana, M. G., D'Aurea, C. V. R., Youngstedt, S. D., Tufik, S. and de Mello, M. T., 2011. Effects of moderate aerobic exercise training on chronic primary insomnia. *Sleep Medicine*, 12(10), pp. 1018–27.

Penedo, F. J. and Dahn, J. R., 2005. Exercise and well-being: a review of mental and physical health benefits associated with physical activity. *Current Opinion in Psychiatry*, 18(2), pp. 189–93.

Twenge, J., Sep. 2017. Have smartphones destroyed a generation? *The Atlantic*. Retrieved from https://www.theatlantic.com/magazine/archive/2017/09/has-the-smartphone-destroyed-a-generation/534198/.

The Drugs Don't Work (At Least Not For Me)

Cipriani, A., Furukawa, T. A., Salanti, G., Chaimani, A., Atkinson, L. Z., Ogawa, Y., Leucht, S., Ruhe, H. G., Turner, E. H., Higgins, J. P. and Egger, M., 2018. Comparative efficacy and acceptability of 21 anti-depressant drugs for the acute treatment of adults with major depressive disorder: a systematic review and network meta-analysis. *Focus*, *16*(4), pp. 420–9.

Healy, D., 2006. *Let Them Eat Prozac: The unhealthy relationship between the pharmaceutical industry and depression*. NYU Press.

Pescosolido, B. A., 2013. The public stigma of mental illness: What do we think; what do we know; what can we prove?. *Journal of Health and Social Behavior*, *54*(1), pp. 1–21.

ACKNOWLEDGEMENTS

THIS BOOK WOULDN'T have been possible without the boundless support, energy and trust of Lauren Whelan, Julia Kellaway and everyone at Yellow Kite. You've taken a punt on me, and I'm very grateful for it.

I'm also extremely grateful for my generous, supportive and endlessly enthusiastic parents. I could tell them I wanted to join the circus and they'd still support me. 'Let's make a plan,' would be my dad's response; 'Great idea! Now, have you seen my scissors?' would be my mum's.

My two brothers, Tom and Benj, have also been a huge source of support throughout all this. As has my cousin-who-is-nearly-a-brother, Will. And my lovely sister-in-law, Gin.

Which is to say nothing of my brilliant mates. Adriana Ciravegna – the best thing to come out of Italy since pasta. Lulu Dillon – Beaconsfield's answer to Rescue Remedy. Tom Spencer – quite the most dependable man on Earth. Pom Beeley – a rock of a mate. As well as Charles Crane, Sophia

Hungerford, Izzy Cumming-Bruce, Harry Parnell, Lucy Rigby, Cosima Glaister, James and Harry Staight, Gemma Hitchens, Flo Fletcher, Livvy Wells, Conor Cadden, Jamie Elder, James Gummer, Nick Mason, Ivan de Klee, Will Brookes, Alice Leahy, John Okell, Dave Kells, Richard Hadler, Natalia Rosek, Nathan Wilson, Grant Chapman, Charlie Bell, Chris Walker, Kat Christian, Jack Yeoman, Sara Hitchens, Harry Linell, Peter Chadlington and Stephen Fry.

I must make a special mention of Olly Cassels and his lovely wife Clem. Not only for allowing me to gatecrash their lives while writing this, but also for putting me on the wiggly road to authorship in the first place.

Thank you also to 'Brian', the man with the plan. I know almost nothing about you or your life, but I do know that you're an unspeakably kind and patient man. And I'm also sure that you saved my life. Thank you.

Finally, then, to Cali. Thank you for loving me, even when I've made it hard to. You're my best mate, the love of my life and I fancy you loads.